Horm

Don't let them

Dr Sandra Cabot

Hormones - Don't Let Them Ruin Your Life
Copyright © 1991 Dr Sandra Cabot

First Published 1991 by WHAS Pty Ltd
Fully Updated and Revised 2004

WHAS Pty Ltd
P. O. Box 689
Camden NSW, 2570 Australia
Phone 02 4655 8855
www.whas.com.au

ISBN: 0 958613761

1. Hormones. 2. Women's Health. 3. Postpartum Depression.
4. Post Natal Depression. 5. Pre-Menstrual Syndrome.
6. Infertility. 7. Sex Drive. 8. Contraception. 9. Sterilisation

Printed by Griffin Press, South Australia
Type set by Hero Productions: 0414 539 419

Dedication

This book is dedicated to my two grandmothers Rosina Adelaide McRae and Suzannah Dalton who were both strong and inspiring women ahead of their time.

About the Author

Dr Sandra Cabot MBBS, DRCOG, is a medical doctor who has extensive clinical experience; she treats patients with hormonal imbalances, chronic diseases and weight problems.

Dr Cabot works with other medical doctors and her team of naturopaths; her practices are situated in Camden and Broadway, Sydney, NSW.

Dr Sandra Cabot began studying nutritional medicine while she was a medical student and has been a pioneer in the area of holistic healing. She graduated in medicine with honours from the University of Adelaide, South Australia in 1975. During the 1980s Dr Cabot worked as a volunteer in the largest missionary Christian hospital in India, tending to the poor indigenous women.

Dr Cabot founded the National Women's Health Advisory Service in 1981, as a non-government funded service. This service has provided telephone and internet advice for women of all ages who want to know all their options.

For more information phone Dr Cabot's Health Line on 02 4655 8855.

Melissa Nash BScDipHM is a clinical nutritionist and she co-authored with Dr Cabot the chapter on Polycystic Ovarian Syndrome.

Dr Cabot pilots herself to many cities and country towns in Australia where she is invited to speak at seminars and exhibitions.

Her free magazine called "Ask Dr Sandra Cabot" is available through health food stores and can also be read on line at www.whas.com.au

FOREWORD

By Dr Oscar Horky MBBS, FRCOG, DGO (Paris), FRACOG

I have followed Dr Sandra Cabot's medical progress over the last 15 years with great interest and increasing admiration. Her understanding of human beings and their ills was apparent from her earliest days in practice. It was my pleasure to be involved in mutually treating patients and to observe her dealing first hand with the sick. She developed a technique of healing the whole person and not just one organ.

Dr Cabot uses the total pharmacopoeia and has proven that modern medicine can and must co-exist with naturopathic therapies. Needless to say, her fame spread to such a degree that she could not possibly attend to all who needed her. A lesser person would have left it at that, but not Dr Cabot. For all those patients she could not personally see, she decided to put her knowledge into helpful books. Her first book titled Women's Health was published in 1987, after which she wrote many more books including The Body Shaping Diet, The Liver Cleansing Diet, Raw Juices can Save your Life, Can't Lose Weight? You could have Syndrome X, and Hormone Replacement Therapy –The Real Truth.

This book deals with the most intricate and complex of all medical subjects: hormones and the endocrine system. A scholarly review of the scientific knowledge has been undertaken and translated into a language that every person can understand. Her personal anecdotes reveal that hormonal dysfunction can adversely affect us all, and more importantly can now be successfully corrected in very many cases.

This book is essential reading for women of all ages and their male partners.

Dr Oscar Horky is a specialist obstetrician and gynaecologist in Western Australia.

CONTENTS

Hormones are beyond a doubt the most powerful chemicals in your body. They have the power to be physically and emotionally shattering or they can make you feel wonderfully alive. No-one wants to live on a series of extreme highs or lows and we don't have to do that anymore because it's now possible to fine-tune your hormones to avoid this "hormonal seesaw". To feel really well most of the time, you need to achieve a balance in your hormones and this book teaches you how. Many women feel confused and somewhat helpless and, as victims of their hormones, are desperately searching for ways to escape the prison of hormonal chaos.

Why are hormonal imbalances more common these days?

The incidence of hormonal disorders in women has increased over the last 20 years mainly because of sociological, environmental and dietary factors. *We are seeing a higher incidence of hormonal imbalances such as –*

- Precocious puberty
- Polycystic Ovarian Syndrome
- Unexplained infertility
- Endometriosis
- Irregular menstrual cycles
- Premenstrual syndrome
- Premature ovarian decline
- Syndrome X – the chemical imbalance of insulin resistance which leads to excess weight gain

These hormonal disorders reduce the quality of women's lives and need to be addressed at a deeper level, where we are not just treating the symptoms of these problems.

Why are hormonal imbalances more common?

1. Women have fewer children and have children later in life, which leads to a relative deficiency of the hormone progesterone

2. The chemicals we are exposed to in this toxic day and age. Most of these chemicals were developed during and subsequent to the industrial boom after World War II. These chemicals are capable of disrupting the function of the endocrine glands and are known as "endocrine disruptors". They are able to attach to hormone receptors on the cell membranes and can block the action of our own naturally produced hormones. These chemicals include pesticides, plastics, polychlorinated biphenyls (PCBs) and solvents. They pollute the air, water ways and

food chain and are found in many household products. We willingly and sometimes unwittingly ingest artificial chemicals such as MSG and aspartame in diet sodas and diet foods. These are known as excito-toxins because they overstimulate the nervous system causing disruptions in the hypothalamus and pancreas. This disrupts the endocrine glands and increases the risk of obesity.

3. Dietary imbalances – we consume too much carbohydrate from refined flour products and sugar, which increases our insulin levels causing weight gain and ovarian dysfunction. We consume too much unhealthy fat from hydrogenated oils and deep fried food. It is healthier to avoid the fatty parts of meat, as these often accumulate fat-soluble toxic chemicals, so trim off the fat and remove the skin from poultry (unless it's organic). Deep fried foods are unhealthy because the fat becomes oxidised producing free radicals, which can damage the liver and endocrine glands. Hormonal imbalances can be greatly improved by food combining and detoxification of the body – for more information see www.liverdoctor.com and the book titled "*The Liver Cleansing Diet.*"

In this book we will look at how hormones affect your mental and emotional state, your nerves, sexuality, skin, hair, body weight and shape, ageing, the menstrual cycle, headaches and your energy. We will resolve your dilemmas about the oral contraceptive pill and tubal ligation.

This is a "save your life book" and gives you the tools to communicate effectively with your own doctor and to work with your doctor to gain control of your hormones. With the increased self understanding that you will acquire from this book you will have the confidence to be assertive with your health care providers to demand the type and quality of care that you need. Balancing your hormones naturally will free you to realise your full potential and enjoy good health. With the right information, you need not let your hormones ruin your life.

I work with a team of doctors and naturopaths in Sydney and also keep a data base of an Australia-wide network of doctors who believe in the technique of natural hormone balancing. You may phone the Women's Health Advisory Service for more information (0246558855) and also visit us online where you will find our newsletters and helpful naturopaths to whom you can email your questions. You will also find information about our clinics – at www.whas.com.au. As I have always said- "Hormones make the world go round!" We hope you like our little hormone devil on the back cover of this book!

Dr Sandra Cabot

CHAPTER 1

What is a Hormone?

Hormones are body chemicals that carry messages from one part of the body to another. They are manufactured in specialised glands (endocrine glands) located in various places in our body and are circulated in the blood stream to body cells where their presence makes a dramatic impact. (See Diagram 1).

Some examples of the many glands required to keep our cells functioning in harmony are:

- The thyroid gland, which manufactures thyroid hormone
- The adrenal glands, which manufacture adrenalin, cortisol, DHEA and other steroid hormones
- The ovaries, which produce the sex hormones oestrogen and progesterone
- The pituitary gland which manufactures hormones that control other glands

Compared to many other body chemicals, hormones are relatively slow acting in producing their effects upon our cells. Hormones determine the rate at which our cells burn up food substances and release energy and thus control the metabolic rate – this is of great importance to those who battle with a weight problem! Hormones also determine what metabolic products our cells will produce such as milk, hair, secretions or enzymes.

Hormones are extremely potent molecules and in some cases, less than one millionth of a gram is enough to trigger their effects. They are far too small to be seen even under a microscope. After they have completed their tasks, hormones are broken down by the cells themselves or are carried to the liver for breakdown. They are then either excreted from the body via the bile or urine or are used again to manufacture new hormone molecules.

Hormones can be likened to chemical keys that turn vitally important metabolic locks in our cells. The turning of these locks stimulates activity within the cells of our brain, intestines, muscles, genital organs and skin. Indeed all our cells are influenced to some degree by these amazing hormonal keys. (See Diagram 2).

Without hormonal keys, the metabolic locks on our cells remain closed and the full potential of our cells is not realised. This could be compared to a corporation where the employees are unable to communicate with the managing director and are left to do their own thing. Such a corporation would lack any unified direction or growth and result in chaos. This is precisely what happens in our cells without the correct type and balance of hormones.

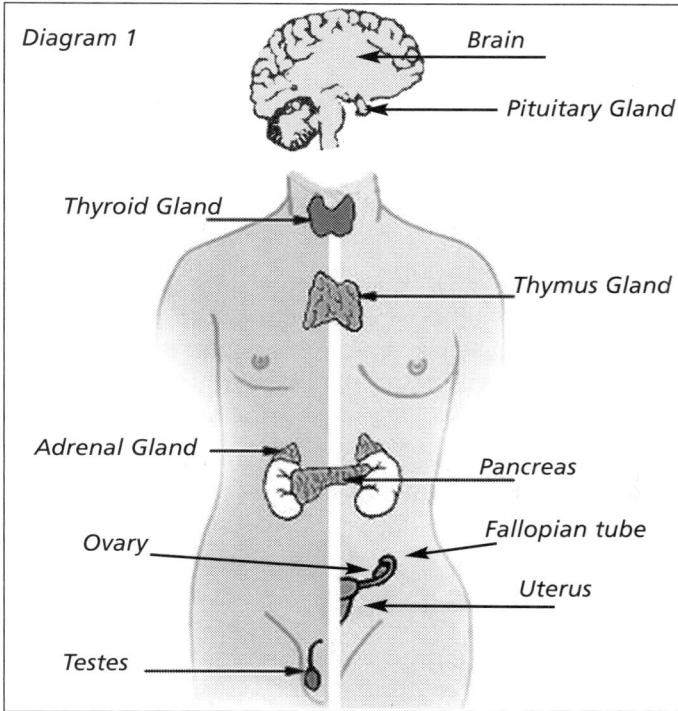

Diagram 1

Brain
Pituitary Gland
Thyroid Gland
Thymus Gland
Adrenal Gland
Pancreas
Ovary
Fallopian tube
Uterus
Testes

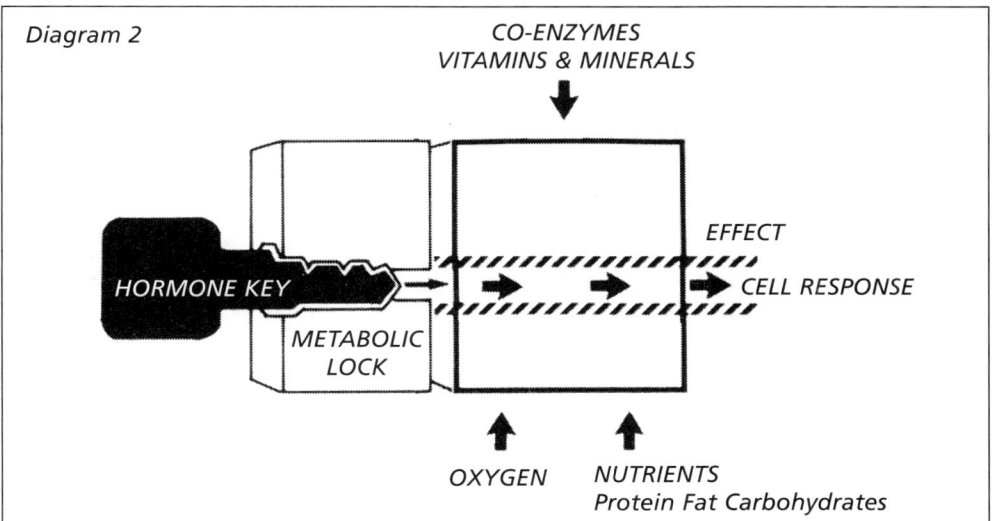

Diagram 2

CO-ENZYMES
VITAMINS & MINERALS

HORMONE KEY

METABOLIC LOCK

EFFECT
CELL RESPONSE

OXYGEN   NUTRIENTS
Protein Fat Carbohydrates

CHAPTER 2

The Pre-Menstrual Syndrome

Katrina had married at the age of 19 against the advice of parents and friends. By the age of 22, she had two beautiful toddlers and a successful husband, who doted on his children. Katrina should have been blissfully happy, but she wasn't. For two weeks before her periods, she became morose, irritable and hurtful to her family. She lost interest in sex and felt ugly and unloved.

When her menstrual flow began, the dark clouds dissolved and she became her carefree self again but with bitter memories of how she had hurt those she loved. She became the caring mother and wife and resumed her painting and pottery, as an expression of her creative spirit. Life was good again until ovulation began and then, with monotonous regularity, the dark storm clouds gathered around.

Bettina, aged 37 had a vastly different lifestyle to Katrina. She was the typical career woman, an executive in a multi-national corporation. She told her friends that she had simply forgotten to have children and marriage was not on her agenda in the context of her sixty-five hour working week. There were many who envied her but underneath her cool executive veneer, Bettina was starting to crack. She jumped down the throats of her colleagues, mixed up appointments and became confused for about seven days before each period. She made obvious and serious mistakes and blamed others for not covering up for her inadequacies. The only way Bettina could cope during the week before her period was by drinking more alcohol and chain-smoking. She was wracked by intense headaches for three days before every period and needed frequent doses of painkillers to keep going. As soon as her period began, her headaches vanished and she became once again the cool, calm, collected executive with the seemingly perfect veneer. Deep down, Bettina knew that if this monthly imbalance continued, she would burn out by the age of 45.

Perhaps you can see yourself in these two very different women. As a doctor, I see hundreds of such cases in my surgery every year. It is the classic, woeful tale of Pre-menstrual Syndrome or PMS. Most women will have heard of PMS, as it has received extensive coverage in the press and media, but it still remains a very misunderstood and poorly treated issue.

PMS is surprisingly common and surprisingly variable. About 50% of women in their reproductive years will notice unpleasant mental and physical changes in themselves sometime during the two weeks before the menstrual bleeding begins.

PMS is the medical term used to describe the collection of different mental and physical problems that may occur during the second half of the menstrual cycle. There are many different possible symptoms and the important clue is not their nature but the cyclical timing of the symptoms. If the symptoms are due to PMS, they will begin in the second half of the monthly menstrual cycle, sometime after ovulation, and will disappear once the menstrual flow begins. The symptoms will then reappear after ovulation occurs in the next menstrual cycle and so the cyclical repetitive nature of PMS will become apparent. (See Diagram 3). Some women will notice symptoms for the full two weeks preceding bleeding, while others will feel unwell for only several days before bleeding. Some months may be worse than others with a variation in the intensity and type of symptoms.

There are many possible symptoms of PMS and indeed Dr Katharina Dalton, a world authority on this subject, has identified 150 of them. Once again, it is not the type of symptoms but the cyclical relationship of the symptoms before menstrual bleeding that distinguishes PMS from other medical disorders. (Ref 3)

Common Symptoms of the Pre-Menstrual Syndrome

Mental and Psychological

Depression, anxiety, irritability, sudden mood changes, aggression, hostility, alcoholic bouts, drug abuse, panic attacks, insomnia, fatigue, sleepiness, confusion, low self-esteem, paranoia, reduced concentration,

DIAGRAM 3 - THE PMS ROLLER COASTER

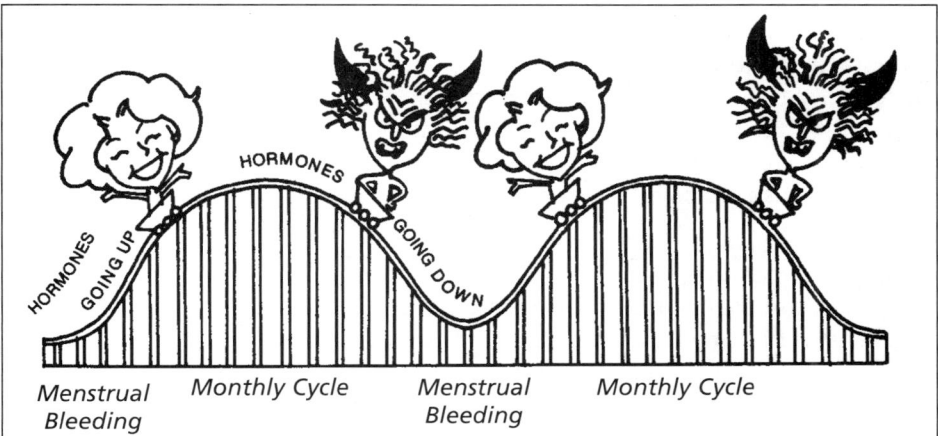

exhaustion, changes in libido. Aggravation of manic depression or obsessive compulsive disorder may occur pre-menstrually and be relieved by the onset of the menstrual blood flow. Some of the more curious symptoms include creative urges or feeling "spaced out."

Physical

Headaches, breast swelling and tenderness, fluid retention, bloating, low blood sugar, food cravings, sugar binges, dramatic changes in weight, clumsiness, poor co-ordination, fainting, acne, general aches and pains, backaches, muscle tension and spasm, constipation and pelvic pain.

Another curious phenomenon is that of "pre-menstrual magnification." This means that medical problems, such as allergies, mouth ulcers, genital herpes, cold sores, candida, asthma, epilepsy, schizophrenia, arthritis, migraine, etc, may become worse during the two pre-menstrual weeks. During this time, there seems to be a reduction in the general resistance and efficiency of several body systems. If you have an Achilles' heel, it is most likely to affect you in the pre-menstrual zone.

What causes the Pre-Menstrual Syndrome?

I well remember one evening in the country town of Grafton, NSW, relating Hippocrates theory on the causation of female hormonal imbalances to an entirely male audience. These men had come to listen to my after-dinner talk about "How to be a perfect husband". My mother had got me into this rather sticky situation, as she had delighted in 'setting me up' when the male dominated Lions Club had requested my services as an after-dinner speaker.

As I explained that Hippocrates had blamed a "wandering uterus" that travelled up to the brain and disturbed the emotions, a little man at the front of the audience became wide-eyed and intrigued. I further related that Hippocrates' treatment for PMS was to entice the wayward uterus back into its rightful position in the pelvis by burning aromatic incense at the vaginal opening. At this juncture, the same man's jaw fell open and he looked relieved. After my light-hearted dissertation, he came up to me and whispered in my ear saying that "he had problems at home and did I have any of that incense for sale!" It is amazing what desperate husbands will do!

After the Hippocrates treatment, it took until 1931 for doctors to realise that hormones had something to do with PMS! A certain Dr Franks preached the theory that too much oestrogen caused PMS. His treatment was even more drastic than that of Hippocrates, as he recommended large doses of laxatives to flush the demon hormones out of the body. Dr Franks claimed great success with this treatment, which is little wonder, as the vio-

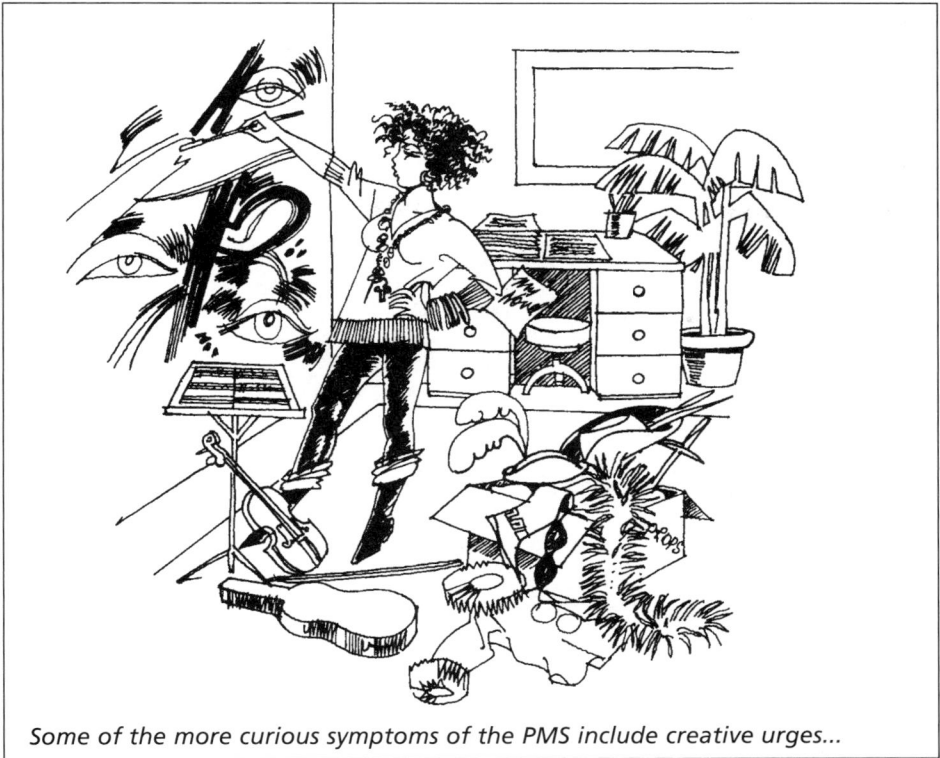

Some of the more curious symptoms of the PMS include creative urges...

lence of the resulting diarrhoea was enough to drown out all the other woes of the PMS victim.

Some women even had their ovaries subjected to radiation and consequent destruction in a desperate attempt to end their PMS.

There is no doubt that the monthly cyclical fluctuations in the levels of the sex hormones oestrogen and progesterone play a large role in causing PMS. This is supported by the observation that PMS begins only after puberty, recurs on a monthly basis and disappears during pregnancy and after the menopause.

If you glance at Diagram 4, you will see the mushroom-shaped pituitary gland situated at the base of the brain. The pituitary gland controls and "speaks" to the ovaries by sending chemical messengers called Follicle Stimulating Hormone (FSH) and Luteinizing Hormones (LH) via the blood stream to the ovaries. FSH and LH stimulate the ovaries to manufacture both oestrogen and progesterone.

Ovulation occurs when an ovary releases a mature egg and the cells left

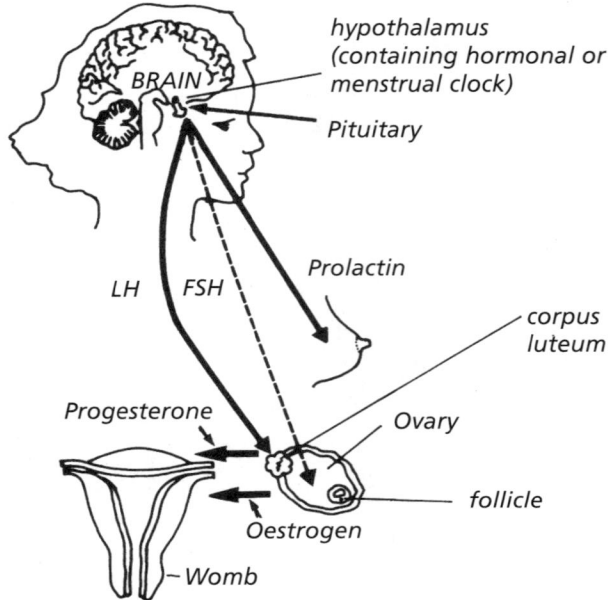

DIAGRAM 4

hypothalamus (containing hormonal or menstrual clock)

Pituitary

BRAIN

Prolactin

LH FSH

corpus luteum

Progesterone

Ovary

follicle

Oestrogen

Womb

behind in the ovary then form a small yellow coloured gland called the corpus luteum. For the 2 weeks after ovulation the corpus luteum manufactures the hormone progesterone and if it is healthy it manufactures sufficient amounts of this wonderful health promoting hormone (Diagram 5).

It is after ovulation in PMS sufferers that the fireworks begin. In a woman without PMS, the levels of oestrogen and progesterone remain in sufficient and balanced amounts between ovulation and menstrual bleeding. In a woman with PMS, the levels of oestrogen and progesterone are out of balance with insufficient oestrogen and/or progesterone between ovulation and bleeding. (Diagram 6).

Some researchers believe that it is the ratio of oestrogen to progesterone that is more important than the absolute amounts of these hormones. They have found that women, who have too much oestrogen compared to progesterone (oestrogen dominance), have anxiety and tension. Women with too little oestrogen compared to progesterone complain of depression during the pre-menstrual phase.

Indeed, there are many subtle variations in the levels of sex hormones produced from the ovaries and a whole range of imbalances in all three ovarian sex hormones, oestrogen, progesterone and testosterone can be involved. This accounts for the variation in PMS symptoms between different women and between different cycles in the same woman.

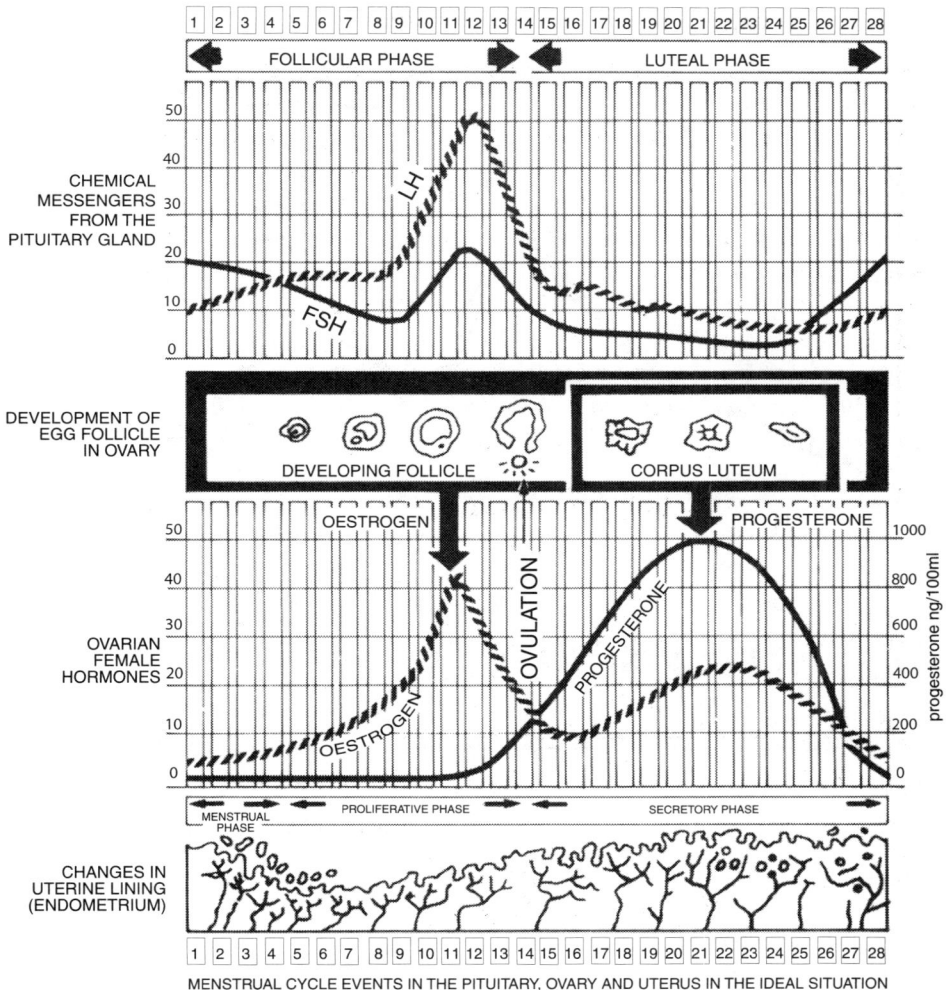

DIAGRAM 5

THE PRE-MENSTRUAL SYNDROME

MENSTRUAL CYCLE EVENTS IN THE PITUITARY, OVARY AND UTERUS IN THE IDEAL SITUATION

FSH = Follicle Stimulating Hormone
LH = Luteinising Hormone

The study of the female sex hormones is called gynaecological endocrinology and it is a relatively new medical specialty with still much to explore. We stand at the frontier of an explosion in the scientific discovery of how imbalances in sex hormones influence our mind and bodies. PMS is truly a Pandora's Box and we have now dared to lift the lid so that one by one, the hormonal demons will be tamed and controlled.

DIAGRAM 6

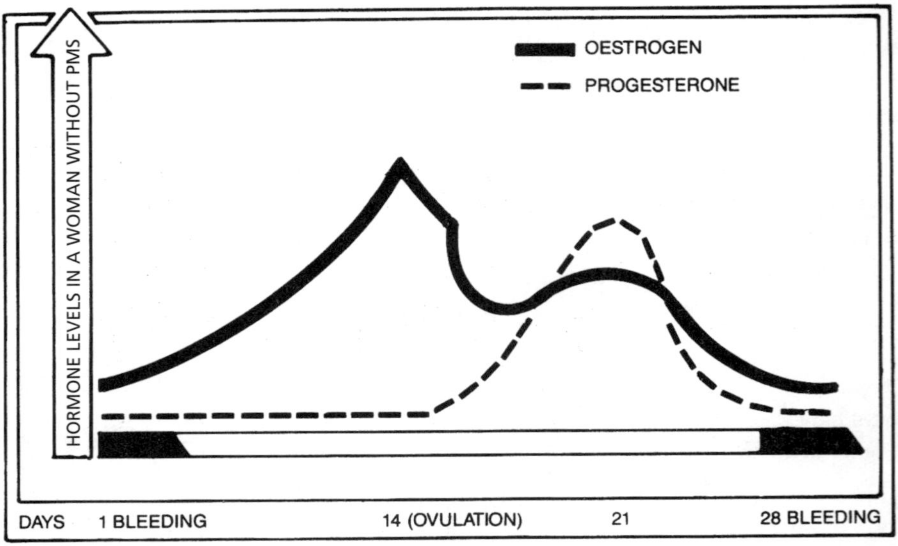
HORMONE LEVELS IN A WOMAN WITHOUT PMS
OESTROGEN
PROGESTERONE
DAYS
1 BLEEDING
14 (OVULATION)
21
28 BLEEDING

NORMAL MENSTRUAL CYCLE — WITHOUT PMS

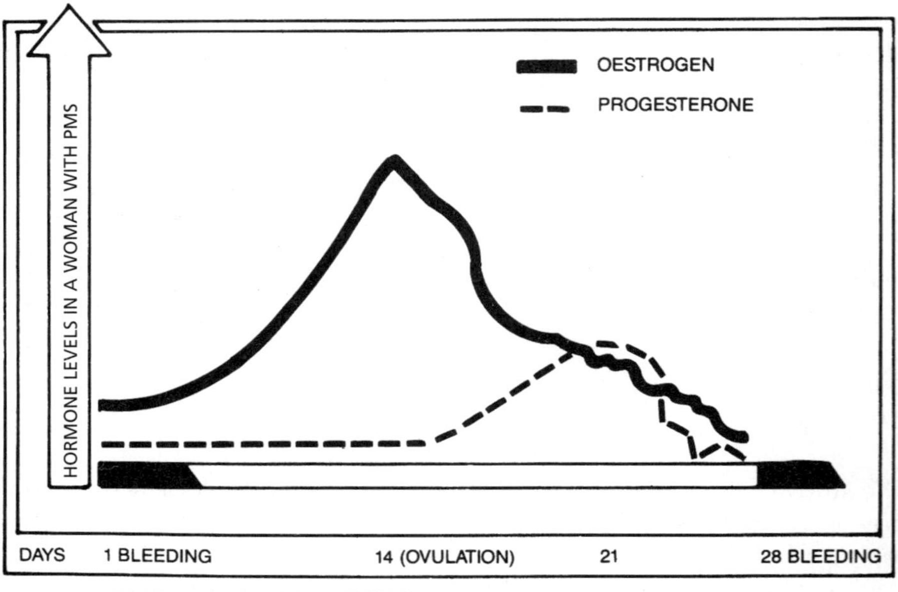
HORMONE LEVELS IN A WOMAN WITH PMS
OESTROGEN
PROGESTERONE
DAYS
1 BLEEDING
14 (OVULATION)
21
28 BLEEDING

PMS MENSTRUAL CYCLE PMS ZONE

Does Nutrition play a role in PMS?

Nutritional imbalances and deficiencies can greatly worsen PMS. I have observed that many women obtain complete relief from PMS after improving their diet and/or taking nutritional supplements. You may, as I did originally, find it surprising that such simple and safe nutritional strategies can completely overcome the sometimes dramatic and severe symptoms of hormonal imbalance and yet, it is a demonstrated fact that I have seen countless times.

Can nutritional supplements help overcome PMS?

A number of studies have found that vitamin B6 in a daily dosage of 25mg to 100mg can give satisfactory relief of many PMS symptoms such as pre-menstrual headaches, fluid retention, irritability and depression in around 60% to 80% of women. (Ref 7,8,9).

Vitamin B6 helps to regulate the brain's biochemistry and is necessary for the conversion of tryptophan to the brain hormone, serotonin.

Serotonin is a natural regulator of mood, sex drive, sleep and appetite. In my experience, vitamin B6 is much more effective if it is taken along with other B complex vitamins, such as vitamin B1 (thiamine), vitamin B2 (riboflavine), vitamin B3 (niacinamide), and vitamin B 5 (pantothenic acid).

I had the pleasure of discussing women's health with the remarkable doctor, Lady Cilento, shortly before her death and she told me that she had had great success in alleviating PMS in thousands of women with one injection every four weeks of vitamin B12 (cyanocobalamin).

This certainly has merit in women with poor diets, heavy menstrual bleeding or in those who are strict vegetarians or suffer with digestive complaints.

One of the anti-oxidants, vitamin E can also be most helpful because it is involved in the production of various hormones from the adrenal and pituitary glands, as well as the vitally important male hormones. Vitamin E is a superb antioxidant protecting the fatty membranes of our cells thereby improving ovarian function and reducing inflammation. Several studies have found it successful in relieving pre-menstrual breast pain and lumpiness. (Ref 10,11).

Zinc and Selenium

Zinc & selenium play a vital role in human metabolism and have been found to be commonly deficient in the diets of western women in the reproductive age group. Zinc and selenium are necessary for proper function of the ovaries, and a healthy immune system and they promote strong and healthy skin and hair. They could be considered minerals to enhance physical beauty and many PMS sufferers should take a regular supplement containing these minerals. Selenium is able to reduce the symptoms of fibrocystic breast disease and has proven anti-cancer properties. (Ref 39)

Magnesium

This mineral is often deficient in women, who consume a diet that is high in refined carbohydrate and sugar. Such a diet will deplete the body of the minerals chromium, manganese, zinc and magnesium and the B complex vitamins. Women with PMS have been found to have lower levels of magnesium in their red blood cells, compared to PMS-free women. (Ref 12). Women with a magnesium deficiency often crave sugar and in particular, chocolate, which is a source of dietary magnesium, albeit a poor one. I have found that many chocoholics can easily resist chocolate binges after commencing a magnesium supplement. Magnesium deficiency will also predispose you to muscular cramps, palpitations, anxiety, insomnia and headaches. In particular migraine headaches can be helped greatly by taking a high dose magnesium supplement.

Other important minerals that help to relieve PMS symptoms are calcium, chromium, manganese and iron. These are helpful for women with fatigue and unstable blood sugar levels, which cause mood changes, light-headedness and sugar cravings, particularly if a meal is missed.

TABLE 2

Foods	Essential Fatty Acids	Prostaglandin Family	Effect in Body
Sesame and sunflower seeds and their oils,cold pressed vegetable oils, blackcurrant seed oil, evening primrose oil and borage oil	Linoleic acid, Gamma linolenic acid	Prostaglandin 1 (desirable)	Reduces pain and inflammation
Fatty or preserved meats, full-cream dairy products, deep fried foods, processed foods and take-away meals	Arachidonic acid	Prostaglandin 2 (undesirable)	Increases pain and inflammation; can result in sticky platelets and poor circulation
Flaxseed (linseed) oil, blackcurrant seeds and their oil, fish oil, mackeral and fresh fish (from cold deep oceans) sardines, tuna, salmon (must not be fried)	Alpha linolenic acid, Eicosapentaenoic acid (EPA)	Prostaglandin 3 (desirable)	Reduces pain and inflammation

A multivitamin & mineral tablet containing iron should be taken by all women with heavy menstrual bleeding.

A suitable brand of woman's multi is called Power Woman and it contains all of the vitamins and minerals discussed in this section. Power Woman multi also contains female balancing herbs which have been used traditionally to help women with hormonal imbalances. The dosage of Power Woman is one tablet daily so it works out to be very economical.

Essential Fatty Acids

The dietary essential fatty acids are the building blocks for a very powerful group of hormone-like chemicals in our body called "prostaglandins". Prostaglandins regulate many vital body functions such as hormone production, circulation, immune function and inflammation, just to name a few. It is helpful for you to know that there are three different families of prostaglandins and the prostaglandin 2 family promotes inflammation and pain, whereas the prostaglandin 1 and prostaglandin 3 families reduce inflammation and pain. (At least, it's 2 to 1 in favour of the good guys). See Table 2 to see what foods provide you with certain essential fatty acids, which in turn are used to manufacture prostaglandins in your body.

Doctors frequently prescribe the powerful anti-prostaglandin drugs also known as non-steroidal anti-inflammatory drugs (NSAIDs). These NSAIDs suppress production in the body of all three families of prostaglandins (good and bad alike) and that is why there are sometimes side effects from these drugs. Examples of these drugs are Indocid, Naprogesic and Ponstan and they can be very effective in stopping the pain and inflammation of headaches, arthritis and period pains.

I have found that in many cases of PMS, headaches or period periods, it is possible to rebalance the three prostaglandin families simply by changing the diet and taking supplements of essential fatty acids. This reduces pain and inflammation in a natural way.

To reduce the amounts of the undesirable prostaglandin 2 family you should reduce your intake of saturated fats, fatty meats and fried food.

To increase the production of the desirable prostaglandin 1 and prostaglandin 3 families, you should consume a diet that is high in raw seeds, sprouts, raw nuts, vegetables, fish and cold pressed seed & vegetable oils. (Table 2)

Another efficient way to balance the prostaglandin families is to take supplements of essential fatty acids. The best known one is evening primrose oil (EPO) which contains the essential fatty acids linoleic acid and gamma linolenic acid (GLA). GLA can be hard to come by in a normal western diet, the highest source being found in breast milk, which partly explains why breast-fed babies are generally healthier than bottle-fed babies. EPO will increase the prostaglandin 1 family and can be remarkably effective in reducing pre-menstrual headaches, arthritis, breast tenderness, period pains and other symptoms of PMS. EPO is helpful for ovarian function and helps to return regularity to the menstrual cycle and reduces ovarian cysts.

My sister, Madeleine, an actress, finds capsules containing a combination of flaxseed oil and evening primrose oil superb for her hair and skin, and says that she is happy to go without several of life's little luxuries provided she can have her capsules of "Flaxseed Plus".

GOLDEN RULES	GOOD EFFECTS
Avoid refined carbohydrates, soft drinks and refined sugars. Get your sugar from fresh fruits.	Aids weight control, stabilises blood sugar levels.
Reduce saturated fats, eg fatty meats, sausages, preserved meats or deep-fried foods, processed and take away meals & some dairy products (such as butter, cream & ice cream)	Aids weight control, reduces hormonal imbalances, reduces cysts in the breast and ovaries, reduces the risk of cancer and reduces inflammation and pain.
Reduce caffine, chocolate and alcohol. Sugar can be replaced with the natural herbal sweetener Stevia	Reduces anxiety and mood changes, fluid retention, headaches and breast pain and breast cysts.
Increase foods high in magnesium and iron, eg whole grains, green leafy vegetables, beetroot, unprocessed cereals, legumes, nuts, seeds, seafood and lean fresh red meat (not essential if you are vegetarian) Culinary seaweeds (such as kelp, arame, dulse, wakame) are excellent sources of trace minerals and calcium. These seaweeds or sea vegetables can be used in soups, stir fries or salads	Reduces headaches and increases energy levels. Prevents iron deficiency anaemia. Increases bone density. Seaweeds reduce body toxicity. Supports the function of the thyroid gland.
Eat 3 meals daily containing first class protein, eg organic eggs, organic poultry, seafood, lean fresh meat and whey protein powder such as Synd-X Slimming Protein Powder, Feta or parmesan cheese provides high quality protein and calcium. An excellent source of first class protein and fibre is obtained by combining 3 of the following at one meal - grains, nuts, seeds & legumes.	Stabilises blood sugar levels, prevents sugar and junk food binges, and increases energy levels. Reduces insulin resistance (Syndrome X) thus aiding weight loss by enhancing fat burning.
Consume foods high in phyto-estrogens such as legumes, whole ground flaxseed and sprouts	Reduces hormonal imbalances and reduces the risk of hormone dependent cancers
Consume foods high inorganic sulphur such as the cruciferous vegetables (broccoli, cauliflower, Brussels sprouts, cabbage, kale, bok choy) and the onion family (onions of all types, leeks, garlic) and organic eggs.	The sulphur in these foods supports the detoxification pathways in the liver which break down excess levels of oestrogens and toxic chemicals that increase hormonal imbalances.

Supplements of fish oil, flaxseed oil and blackcurrant seed oil will increase the production of the desirable prostaglandin 3 family, which is helpful in reducing many PMS type symptoms. (Table 2).

The Anti PMS Diet – Golden Rules

There are a few golden rules to follow and if you observe them six days a week, you will be able to enjoy the occasional indiscretion with impunity and a clear conscience.

Can Lifestyle Changes help PMS?

A reasonably healthy lifestyle is a must if you are serious about beating PMS. Let's check out the benefits of some good habits.

The tools of a healthy diet, lifestyle and nutritional supplements will provide relief for the vast majority of women with mild to moderate PMS. Patience and persistence are vital, as with most types of nutritional medicine, there is a time lapse of six to eight weeks before major improvements are attained.

What Risk Factors Increase Your Chance of PMS?

1. Family History

You won't thank your ancestors for this familial trait but there is no doubt that if your mother, sisters or maternal or paternal grandmother

LIFESTYLE	BENEFITS
A regular exercise program, including some aerobic exercise, some muscle building and relaxing exercises (stretching, yoga, tai-chi)	Reduces muscle spasm and tension. Increases brain endorphins, which are natural euphoric substances. Improves the blood supply to the hormonal glands.
Quit smoking	Nicotine constricts blood vessels and reduces the blood supply to the hormonal glands, brain and the skin. Giving up smoking will increase the hormone output from your ovaries, thus slowing down the ageing process.
Increase water intake to 2-3 litres daily and make yourself raw vegetable and fruit juices.	Aids weight control and reduces headaches. Greatly improves the condition of the skin and hair. Reduces breast pain. Increases energy levels and improves mental clarity and memory.
Reduce alcohol intake especially during the two pre-menstrual weeks.	Avoids embarrassing moments. There is a reduced tolerance to alcohol pre-menstrually with higher blood alcohol levels being attained quickly. Your moods will be much better and far more stable bringing greater self control.

or great-grandmothers had PMS, then you are also more prone to suffer with PMS.

2. Hormonal Triggers

Many women first notice PMS after stopping the oral contraceptive pill, after pregnancy, postnatal depression or miscarriage, after hysterectomy with conservation of the ovaries or after a tubal ligation (surgical sterilisation).

Some women get PMS type symptoms while taking the oral contraceptive pill (OCP) presumably because the synthetic progesterone in the OCP reduces the production of natural progesterone from the ovaries.

3. Stress

PMS may appear for the first time or become much worse after severe or prolonged stress, such as relationship difficulties, financial problems or unwanted pregnancies.

4. Increasing Age

Typically PMS worsens during the 30s, peaking in the mid to late 30s. During the 40s, PMS becomes intertwined with the hormonal deficiencies characteristic of the pre-menopausal years when more severe deficiencies and/or imbalances of oestrogen and progesterone can occur.

5. Being a 21st Century Woman

Today's woman has, on average, two children and spends the rest of her life having regular menstrual cycles with approximately 350 to 400 menstrual periods in her reproductive life span. Therefore, if she is susceptible, she could have 350 to 400 episodes of PMS in her lifetime. Before contraception was available, a woman had around ten pregnancies, each followed by one to two years of breast-feeding. Our great grandmothers usually only menstruated for two to five years out of their whole life span. Thus, as far as Mother Nature is concerned, it would seem that women are not meant to have periods and PMS, and that they are indeed designed to have more pregnancies. Biologically we are meant to be "pregnant and barefoot in the kitchen" but sociologically those days are gone for good! The price we pay is that of progesterone deficiency.

Is there a Test for PMS?

The most accurate way to determine if you have PMS is to keep a menstrual calendar on which you chart the timing of your symptoms and menstrual bleeding. It is not the type of symptoms that is important, but rather the fact that your symptoms recur every month, some time after ovulation. These symptoms are relieved when menstrual bleeding is established.

The chart of Maggie (Page 27) illustrates a classic tale of PMS and there is a chart for you to photocopy and use to write your own symptoms on (see Page 26). Keep your chart accurately for three months and then take it along to your doctor to enable a correct diagnosis of your hormonal imbalance.

Generally speaking, blood and/or salivary tests to measure hormone levels are not necessary, but if your doctor is unsure of the diagnosis, or if a serious hormonal imbalance is suspected, then tests are vitally important. It is best to measure the hormone levels in the blood or saliva when you feel at your worst, as determined by your menstrual calendar. This will pinpoint exactly what type of hormonal imbalance you could have.

Your Own Menstrual Calendar (see page 26)

On this chart mark the days of menstrual bleeding with an 'M' and the days of your MOST IMPORTANT SYMPTOMS with an appropriate symbol, eg:

H = headache
B = bloatedness/water retention
BT = breast tenderness
D = depression
I = irritability
P = period pains
or invent symbols for your priority symptoms. Even if you are not menstruating, eg have had a hysterectomy, it will help your doctor if you chart the dates of your symptoms.

The Story of Paula

In its most severe manifestation, the pre-menstrual syndrome is a disorder that can ruin your life. This was brought home to me one day by a 42-year old librarian called Paula, who came to see me as her last hope. Paula had first noticed severe mood changes before menstruation, shortly after an early puberty at the age of 10. By the age of 18, her pre-menstrual depression was so severe that she attempted suicide with an overdose of her mother's sedatives. She was diagnosed as manic-depressive and prescribed the drug Lithium. This reduced her mood swings but she still felt unwell with headaches, bloating, sore breasts and extreme fatigue for ten days before her menstrual bleeding. Paula was gradually taken off Lithium so that she could

	Jan	Feb	Mar	Apr	May	Jun	Jul	Aug	Sep	Oct	Nov	Dec
1												
2												
3												
4												
5												
6												
7												
8												
9												
10												
11												
12												
13												
14												
15												
16												
17												
18												
19												
20												
21												
22												
23												
24												
25												
26												
27												
28												
29												
30												
31												

MAGGIE'S CHART

	JANUARY	FEBRUARY	MARCH	APRIL
1		H B D	M	
2	B	M P	M	
3	B	M P	M	
4	B	M		
5	H B D	M		
6	H B D	M		
7	H B D			
8	M P			
9	M P			
10	M			
11	M			
12	M			D
13				B D
14				B D
15				B D
16				B D
17				H B D
18				M P
19			D	M
20			B D	M
21			B D	M
22		D	H B D	M
23		B D	H B D	
24		H B D	M P	
25		H B D	M P	
26		H B D	M	
27	B	M P	M	
28	B	M	M	
29	B D			
30	H B D			
31	H B D			

CODE for Maggie's Chart

M = Menstrual Bleeding   B = Breast Pain

D = depression   P = Period Pain

H = Headaches

Maggie has a 5 day bleeding cycle approximately every 25 days.

become pregnant and by the third month of her pregnancy, she felt wonderful. She said "For the first time in my life, I feel in control, peaceful and free of headaches and I love the feeling of those huge amounts of hormones filling up my body". Paula had a natural birth and things were going well until six weeks after childbirth, when severe postnatal depression began. Paula again attempted suicide and was again prescribed Lithium. Twelve months later at the age of 31, Paula, terrified of another episode of postnatal depression, begged for sterilisation by having her tubes tied (tubal ligation). After consulting six gynaecologists, the tubal ligation was unfortunately performed and, not surprisingly, she then began to experience severe PMS. For twelve days before every period, she felt dead and found herself in a deep pit of depression and anger. Her head ached, her abdomen swelled and she became aggressive with her husband and child. Paula felt trapped knowing that every month after ovulation she would feel as if a switch inside her brain turned on producing volcanic changes in her personality and body. Once her menstrual bleeding started, the switch would be turned off and the depression, aggression and headaches would miraculously vanish. After menstruation she felt in control but was haunted by feelings of remorse and guilt for the disruption she had caused. Her husband could recognise the night and day effect caused by this hormonal switch and he could see that she needed help. Paula visited eight different gynaecologists and tried diuretics, sedatives, anti-depressants, the oral contraceptive pill, synthetic progesterone, psychotherapy and chiropractic treatment. In a desperate attempt to save her marriage, she asked for a hysterectomy and reluctantly, feeling that she had tried all possible therapies, her last doctor removed her uterus.

Paula felt much better for three months after her hysterectomy until during the fourth month she noticed that her depression and anger returned for two weeks. For the next six months, she found that for two weeks out of every four weeks, she was again in the grip of severe mood changes. She returned to the doctor begging to have her ovaries removed. Thankfully, this time the doctor refused and referred her to a psychiatrist.

Paula had classic PMS in a severe degree and was in urgent need of natural hormone therapy. Her hysterectomy had relieved her headaches and fatigue but had done nothing to quell the cyclical surges and falls of sex hormones from her ovaries. She felt great when her ovaries were pumping out oestrogen and progesterone and terrible when they stopped. Paula's case supports the research finding that when the uterus is removed and the ovaries are left in place, the symptoms and hormonal changes of PMS may persist, although often to a lesser degree. (Ref 2).

I suggested to Paula that she would feel more emotionally stable if we maintained a steady and adequate level of the natural oestrogen, oestradiol, and natural progesterone in her blood every day. She willingly accepted an initial course of a lozenge (troche) containing a combination of natural oestradiol and natural progesterone. Two months after commencing the troches, Paula felt stable and happy again and remarked that the constant hormone levels in her blood provided by her troches made her feel the way she felt during pregnancy. Paula could now cope and her daily life was much easier. She felt as if a prison door had been unlocked and she would no longer be trapped in a vicious hormone cycle. Such can be the drama of severe PMS. Women are 'hormonal creatures', riding upon the waves of hormonal surges and indeed this is largely responsible for the alluring mystery that womanhood presents to males. However for a significant percentage of women, the price of this hormonal uniqueness is too much to pay.

Thankfully, we no longer have to be victims of erratic hormonal imbalances as modern day hormonal therapy can re-programme our hormonal cycle. One could say the self-programmable bionic woman has arrived!

Hormonal treatment for PMS

In severe cases of PMS that do not respond to nutritional supplements or anti-depressants, corrective hormonal therapy can be life-saving. If PMS is so severe that it is associated with uncontrollable mood changes, reduced ability to function, thoughts of suicide, marital disruption, child abuse or dangerous behaviour, then hormonal therapy is usually required to restore equanimity. Many of these women have been offered sedatives and counselling and come along to the doctor desperately hoping that hormonal help will be at hand. Thankfully, it is, and it can be dramatically effective.

Progesterone

The use of natural progesterone was first advocated back in the 1970s by Dr Katharina Dalton, an English physician who was somewhat of a 'PMS Guru'. Dr Dalton dedicated her life to helping women with hormonal imbalances and her research and books have shown natural progesterone to be effective in relieving many types of PMS. (Ref 3,4,5).

Natural progesterone can be very useful in reducing the following problems, which may occur, or become much worse, during the pre-menstrual phase of the monthly cycle –

Depression, anxiety, and mood changes
Fatigue and low blood sugar levels
Heavy menstrual bleeding and menstrual pain
Pelvic congestion and bloating
Breast pain, Migraines, Epilepsy, Asthma

It is important to realise that Dr Dalton only recommends the use of natural progesterone, which has a chemical structure identical to the progesterone produced by the ovaries. Natural progesterone is made in the laboratory from the plant hormone called diosgenin found in soybeans and sweet potatoes (yams). Because natural progesterone is identical to the progesterone produced by the ovaries it is called a "bio-identical hormone".

Unfortunately, doctors often prescribe strong synthetic progesterones called 'progestogens' for PMS sufferers, mistakenly believing that they will have the same effect as natural progesterone. This is not true and synthetic progesterone will usually make most of the symptoms of PMS much worse. Many of these synthetic progestogens are derived from male (testosterone-like) synthetic hormones and so may cause side effects such as increased appetite, depression, irritability, weight gain, fluid retention, acne, greasy skin and increased cholesterol. These synthetic progestogen hormones attach onto the natural progesterone receptors found throughout the body and brain, but they cannot switch on all these receptors. Only natural progesterone can turn on ALL the progesterone receptors just as a key turns and releases a lock. So you can understand that synthetic progestogens will not have the same beneficial effect as natural progesterone and indeed many PMS sufferers feel more depressed and tired when they take them. However synthetic progestogens are effective at reducing heavy menstrual bleeding and some types of gynaecological problems.

The progesterone story can be complicated and so I have designed an easy reference table on Pages 34-36 to help you and your doctor understand how to use natural progesterone for PMS. Unfortunately, natural progesterone is not as effective if taken by mouth (orally), as it is destroyed by the liver enzymes after its absorption from the intestines.

Therefore, natural progesterone is best administered by routes that bypass the liver such as

- Creams – which may be rubbed into the skin (transdermal) or inserted high up into the vagina
- Vaginal pessaries or suppositories

Natural progesterone can also be given in the form of lozenges known as "troches", which are NOT designed to be sucked or chewed or swallowed. Theoretically the troche is held between the upper gum and the cheek until it is completely absorbed, with the hormone it contains being transferred directly into the blood stream across the mucous lining of the oral cavity. Natural progesterone can also be administered in the form of capsules which contain tiny (micronised) particles of progesterone. Theoretically these tiny particles of progesterone are more resistant to breakdown by the enzymes in the gut and the liver, so that more progesterone gets into the blood stream.

By giving natural progesterone in these ways, we are aiming to bypass the liver so that the progesterone can be absorbed directly into the circulation and carried to the progesterone receptors on your cells.

As you can see from Table 3 (page 34), the use of progesterone needs to be fine-tuned and should only be administered under regular medical supervision. In general, progesterone is very safe with side effects such as breakthrough bleeding being of nuisance value only. Pure natural progesterone does not cause birth defects or harm to the foetus if you become pregnant, but you should notify your doctor if you are using progesterone while trying to conceive.

Generally natural progesterone therapy is started several days before the expected onset of PMS symptoms and continued daily up to the first day of menstrual bleeding. Once the bleeding starts the progesterone should be stopped. If you find it difficult to judge when to begin using the progesterone, you can start it at the time of ovulation, which is normally 14 days before the expected onset of menstrual bleeding. Each PMS sufferer is an individual and trial and error using different dosages, forms and schedules of progesterone may be required before the symptoms are fully under control. My personal preference is to administer natural progesterone in the form of a cream, which is rubbed into the skin of the inner upper arms or the inner upper thighs. You should apply the cream to dry skin after your shower, and if you shower or bathe twice daily then it may be more effective to apply the cream twice daily after each shower. The cream needs to be rubbed very thoroughly into the skin so that the entire amount is well absorbed into the skin, with no cream remaining visible or detectable on the skin. Some doctors are very cynical about the use of creams containing natural progesterone because they do not believe that the progesterone is effectively absorbed through the skin in to the blood stream. In other words they do not think that clinically effective amounts of progesterone can be achieved in the body by using the creams. However a study published in the American Journal of Obstetrics & Gynaecology in 1999 found that absorption of progesterone from creams was just as good as absorption of oestrogen from patches. They concluded that the application of progesterone cream to the skin appeared to be a safe and effective route of administration.(Ref 13)

Background information on natural progesterone

Progesterone has really been in the limelight lately, with several eminent researchers promoting its benefits.

Progesterone is needed to balance the effects of oestrogen. Oestrogen causes the cells lining the uterus to divide and grow, whereas progesterone inhibits this growth. Oestrogen can be described as a fertiliser, and progesterone as the lawn mower. Thus progesterone is needed to oppose the stimulatory effects of oestrogen on the uterus.

The mechanisms that progesterone uses to keep oestrogen in check are
1. Progesterone reduces the oestrogen receptors stimulating effects upon cancer-promoting genes.
2. Progesterone promotes the conversion of the stronger oestradiol to the weaker type of oestrogen called oestrone.
3. Progesterone reduces the number of oestrogen receptors on the cells, thus reducing the sensitivity of the cells to oestrogen.

These are all very important balancing actions, and this vital role of progesterone explains why all women who are given oestrogen, should always be given progesterone (preferably the natural form), even if they have had a hysterectomy. Natural progesterone is also needed for healthy bone tissue, probably because it stimulates the bone building cells called osteoblasts.

Progesterone is only produced from the ovaries after ovulation. Disorders of ovulation are common, and many women ovulate only irregularly, infrequently or rarely, especially as they approach the pre-menopausal years. The most common cause of infrequent or absent ovulation in pre-menopausal women is Polycystic Ovarian Syndrome. In pre-menopausal women who have ovulation problems, we find that oestrogen is produced from the ovary, but there is no progesterone, or only inadequate amounts of progesterone are produced. The amounts of progesterone are insufficient to balance the oestrogen – this causes the situation of unopposed oestrogen.

This oestrogen will stimulate the lining of the uterus to grow thicker, and the lack of progesterone means that the lining can become abnormally thick – this is called endometrial hyperplasia.

Women with this condition often complain of very heavy menstrual bleeding with large clots. If this hyperplasia becomes chronic, pre-malignant changes may occur in the cells lining the uterus – this is called atypical hyperplasia. Around 20% of women with atypical hyperplasia will go on to get uterine cancer, if this problem is not treated. By administering progesterone (natural or synthetic), we are able to prevent, or even reverse endometrial hyperplasia. Thus progesterone has an anti-cancer effect.

A study published in The Journal of the Climacteric & Postmenopause, Maturitas 20 (1995) 191-198, provides convincing evidence that natural progesterone can control endometrial hyperplasia. In this study, 78 pre-menopausal women with endometrial hyperplasia were treated from the 10th to the 25th day of their menstrual cycle with a vaginal cream containing 100mg of natural micronised progesterone. This progesterone therapy achieved a complete regression (reversal) of the hyperplasia in 90.5% of cases. During treatment there was a significant reduction in the amount, duration and frequency of the menstrual bleeding. Other good news is that minimal side effects were observed during this trial, which is in contrast to synthetic progestogens, which commonly produce side effects.

The researchers concluded that vaginal administration of natural progesterone is –

- Effective in treating hyperplasia
- Safe to use, because it does not exert unfavourable changes on the blood levels of cholesterol

This is in contrast to synthetic progestogens, which may exert adverse changes upon the cholesterol levels.

Thus natural progesterone administered vaginally, should be considered as a serious alternative to synthetic progestogens in clinical practice, especially in women with metabolic disorders such as polycystic ovarian syndrome, Syndrome X, diabetes, hypertension, fatty liver and problems with the levels of blood fats.

Progesterone can also be given in a micronised form (ultrafine consistency), which means that the progesterone particles are much smaller; this is done to improve absorption from the gut. Micronised progesterone is administered in capsules. A dose of 200mg of micronised progesterone, given for 15 days per month, is considered equivalent to 10mg of the synthetic progestogen called Provera. If the natural progesterone is given in a dose of 100mg daily for 25 days per month, this is also considered equivalent to 10mg of Provera. Micronised progesterone was evaluated in the Postmenopausal Estrogen/Progestin Interventions (PEPI) Trial. (Ref 14)

The PEPI Trial showed that 200mg of natural micronised progesterone, given for 12 days of the month, was sufficient to prevent over stimulation of the uterus by Premarin. The micronised progesterone was shown to have a more favourable effect upon blood levels of cholesterol than the synthetic progestogens. Because natural progesterone is more effective in correcting the adverse changes that occur in cholesterol levels after the menopause, it should be safer than synthetic progestogens, when it comes to reducing the risk of heart disease.

The micronised progesterone was found to be as effective as the synthetic progestogens in opposing the effects of oestrogen on the uterus.

Doctors have been educated to use synthetic progestogens in HRT for menopausal women. However now that the WHI study (Ref 15) has shown that synthetic progestogens are not desirable for long term use in HRT, many doctors will be looking towards safer solutions, such as natural prog-

Table 3: PMS Hormone Treatment Chart

HORMONE	TYPE	DOSAGE	BENEFIT	REMEDY FOR SIDE EFFECTS	POSSIBLE SIDE EFFECTS
Natural progesterone	Cream which can be administered via the skin or inserted high up into the vagina last thing at night.	The average dose is 50mg daily but the dose may range from 10mg to 200mg daily. Given for approximately 14 days before the onset of menstrual bleeding.	Relief of the symptoms of the premenstrual syndrome such as mood disorders, pelvic congestion, migraines, heavy bleeding, menstrual pain and fatigue. May reduce breast pain. May increase fertility. May alleviate post natal depression.	Reduce the dose until side effects disappear. Talk to your compounding pharmacist if the cream causes irritation of the skin or vagina, as a different base for the cream can be used.	Some breakthrough bleeding if doses are excessive. Breakthrough bleeding is more likely to occur if the cream is inserted into the vagina. When used vaginally some vaginal irritation may occur if the base of the cream is unsuitable. Excessive doses can lead to bloating and drowsiness.
Natural progesterone	Injections given into the buttocks	25 to 100mg daily given intramuscularly. Given for the 14 days before menstrual bleeding.	Relief of the symptoms of the premenstrual syndrome such as mood disorders, pelvic congestion, migraines, heavy bleeding, menstrual pain and fatigue. May reduce breast pain. May increase fertility. May alleviate post natal depression.	Change to creams or troches of progesterone instead of injections.	The injections are oily so that they act as a slow release depot of progesterone. They may cause tenderness and lumpiness in the buttocks. Some breakthrough bleeding and fluid retention.
Natural progesterone	Troches which are lozenges that are placed between	The average dose is 50mg daily but the dose may range from 25 to	Relief of the symptoms of the premenstrual syndrome such as mood	Reduce the dosage of hormones in the troche, or change to the	If doses are excessive some breakthrough bleeding, drowsiness and fluid retention may occur. In

Type	Form/Description	Dosage	Uses	Alternative	Side effects
	the upper gum and the cheek. They slowly dissolve through the mucous membrane of the cheek and the progesterone is absorbed directly into the circulation. Do not suck, chew or swallow the lozenges. They come in a variety of flavours. Capsules containing micronised progesterone can be swallowed.	200mg daily. Given for the 14 days before menstrual bleeding.	disorders, pelvic congestion, migraines, heavy bleeding, menstrual pain and fatigue. May reduce breast pain. May increase fertility. May alleviate post natal depression	progesterone cream.	some women the troche may produce irritation of the gum. In allergy-prone people the troches may cause allergic type symptoms such as rashes and swelling. The progesterone cream is best used in allergy-prone people. If the troches contain sugar they may increase dental caries.
Semi-natural progesterone called Dydrogesterone (also known as Duphaston). It is a mirror image (retro-isomer) of natural progesterone.	Tablets 10mg	Given in a dose of 5 to 20mg daily for the 14 days before menstrual bleeding.	Reduces heavy painful menstrual bleeding. Useful for reducing endometriosis. May reduce premenstrual mood disorder, although not nearly as effectively as natural progesterone does.	Reduce the dose or change to natural progesterone.	Because it is not entirely natural it may cause some side effects such as weight gain, fluid retention and moodiness. Dydrogesterone is more likely to cause these side effects, as it is not identical to natural progesterone. Some women find it excellent, while others find it ineffective, so some trial and error may be needed.
Synthetic progesterone (also known as progestogens)	Common examples are norethisterone, norgesterol, and medroxy-progesterone acetate tablets.	These tablets can be given every day, or for the 14 days before menstrual bleeding begins. The dosage varies depending upon the brand of tablet and the medical reason for which it is prescribed.	Reduce heavy and/or painful periods. Helpful for endometriosis. May reduce breast tenderness.	Reduce the dose or change to natural progesterone.	These synthetic progestogens have a slightly masculine effect, which may result in weight gain, pimples, greasy skin and hair. Some brands may cause fluid retention, moodiness, depression and elevation of cholesterol. They often make depression and other mood disorders much worse.

HORMONE	TYPE	DOSAGE	BENEFIT	REMEDY FOR SIDE EFFECTS	POSSIBLE SIDE EFFECTS
Natural oestrogen	There are 3 types of natural oestrogen – Oestradiol Oestriol Oestrone Can be given in the form of creams, troches or patches.	Given cyclically for 2 to 3 weeks every month, or used everyday.	May be helpful for mood disorders and may improve libido. Reduces vaginal dryness, discomfort and improves bladder function. Reduces acne and facial hair.	Reduce the dosage of oestrogen, or change to the weakest form of oestrogen which is oestriol. Avoid potent forms of oestrogen such as implants, injections and tablets and use the creams or patches instead. If this does not work, stop the oestrogen and use natural progesterone only.	Excessive doses or the more potent forms of oestrogen can lead to symptoms of oestrogen dominance which include – Breast pain & lumpiness Fluid retention Nausea & gall stones Heavy menstrual bleeding Increased size of fibroids Migraine headaches Aching legs Blood clots Weight gain in the hips & thigh area
Oral Contraceptive Pill (OCP)	There are many types of OCP and the best types for PMS contain the oestrogen called ethinyl-oestradiol combined with a friendly or neutral progestogen such as gestodene or desogestrel.	Can be either a 21 day or 28 day packet of tablets	The OCP can be helpful for PMS but is usually not nearly as effective as natural progesterone. It suppresses ovulation which may help some women with premenstrual mood disorder. The OCP can relieve some types of period pain and reduce heavy bleeding. The OCP provides very good contraception unlike natural progesterone which actually increases fertility in some women!	If you get side effects you will need to experiment with your doctor to try different brands, as they contain different types of hormones. All the hormones used in the OCP are synthetic and some women will be unable to tolerate the side effects.	Migraine headaches which can be severe. Nausea and gall stones. Fluid retention, weight gain and bloating. Reduced or total loss of sex drive. Breast pain and lumpiness. Blood clots and aggravation of varicose veins. Elevation of blood pressure. Moodiness and depression in susceptible women.

Footnote:
Depot = long acting injection lasting for 10 to14 days
Semi-natural progesterone is in between natural and synthetic and is less likely to cause side effects than synthetic progestogens.
It is imperative that women taking drugs or hormones to treat PMS have adequate means of contraception.

esterone. However, natural progesterone does far more than just replace the use of synthetic progestogens, and has several powerful health promoting benefits in itself.

Natural progesterone

- Helps to preserve bone density
- Exerts a favourable effect upon the nervous system
- Exerts an anti-cancer effect against some types of cancer
- Reduces some gynaecological problems such as fibroids and endometriosis.

Natural progesterone has very different effects to synthetic progestogens in the body, and is far less likely to produce unpleasant side effects. Synthetic progestogens can increase the risk of spasm in the coronary arteries, whereas natural progesterone reduces such spasms. Natural progesterone is a smooth muscle relaxant and thus usually helps to reduce menstrual cramps. Synthetic progestogens are far more likely to produce side effects such as weight gain, depression, fluid retention, headaches and breast tenderness.

Jenny Birdsey is a nurse practitioner and counsellor who acts as an advocate and advisor for natural progesterone. Her book is titled "Natural Progesterone - the world's best kept secret"
To speak with Jenny call 03 5222 7145 or visit www.npan.com.au

Oestrogens

In a small number of cases of cyclical premenstrual mood disorder natural progesterone therapy by itself fails to relieve all the symptoms. This is more likely in older women who are pre-menopausal in which case there may be a deficiency of oestrogen as well as progesterone. This can be determined with blood tests (see page 177)

In such cases the use of natural oestrogen combined with the natural progesterone may break the cycle of unpleasant PMS. Some natural oestrogen may also be helpful in PMS sufferers, who have undergone hysterectomy or tubal ligation, as after these operations the blood supply to the ovaries may be reduced. This may result in a reduced hormonal output from the ovaries and therefore increasing PMS.

The types of natural oestrogen that are preferable are

- Oestrogen creams or gels that are rubbed into the skin
- Oestrogen patches

Other types of oestrogen such as oestrogen tablets, oestrogen troches (lozenges) or oestrogen implants and injections can be used, although they are relatively more potent and thus more likely to cause symptoms of oestrogen excess (oestrogen dominance).

Symptoms of oestrogen dominance are
- Breast lumpiness and pain
- Nausea
- Aggravation of gall stones
- Aching legs
- Worsening of varicose veins
- Fluid retention
- Weight gain in the hips & thighs
- Migraine headaches
- Period pains and heavy menstrual bleeding
- Growth of fibroids

The oestrogen implants or injections are best used in women who have had a hysterectomy, as they are relatively potent and may cause an increase in menstrual bleeding and other symptoms of oestrogen dominance. Since the results of the Women's Health Initiative Study (Ref 15) were published in July 2002, all doctors have become aware that long term oestrogen therapy will increase the risk of breast cancer. If the oestrogen is combined with synthetic progesterone this type of hormone therapy becomes even more risky to use long term with an increased risk of blood clots and strokes. Thus it is not wise to use potent forms of oestrogen therapy for many years, and this means that oestrogen implants and injections are really only suitable for short term use. This means for not more than one year.

If you find that you need to take some form of oestrogen to obtain relief from your hormonal symptoms, I suggest that you stick to the oestrogen creams or patches, as the doses used can be much smaller and easily fine tuned to provide the smallest possible dose that relieves your symptoms. It is important to check the results of the hormone therapy with regular blood or salivary levels, and suitable intervals are every 3 months initially and thereafter every 6 to 12 months. If you have your hormone levels tested every month you may have to pay for it yourself, as Medicare may find this excessive.

In my experience I have found that oestrogen implants and/or injections can result in very high blood levels of oestrogen being found on blood tests. This would be worrying if these women decided to continue with these potent forms of oestrogen for many years. In contrast I have found that when using small doses of natural hormones in the form of creams or patches, the blood levels of oestrogen, progesterone and testosterone stay within safe and very modest levels.

Some women find that they only need to use the natural oestrogen during the 14 days preceding menstrual bleeding, whereas others may feel more in balance if they use the oestrogen every day. In women who still have a uterus, the use of natural oestrogen must be balanced with progesterone.

An interesting Case History

Donna aged 43 had first noticed severe PMS eight months after having a tubal ligation (surgical sterilisation). Donna was a top marketing executive with many employees under her supervision and she needed her wits about her every day of the month. She was disgusted by the onset of new and strange hormonal upheavals that she described to me as the 'PMS dichotomy'. Donna found that around the sixteenth day of every menstrual cycle, she felt like two people inside one body – a kind of Dr Jekyll and Mrs Hyde. She described how suddenly she would become irrational and ineffective, while another part of her stood by appalled at what the "PMS self" was doing. She felt out of control until her menstrual bleeding started, and then the two Donnas became one peaceful, together person.

Donna knew that she needed hormone therapy as her mental and emotional changes were severe and her doctor prescribed progesterone pessaries. This only took the edge off her depression and she still felt crazy inside. Donna then began to experience hot flushes and sweating attacks during the week before her menstrual flow. At this time, a blood test confirmed low levels of oestrogen and we recognised that she was approaching her menopause and that her mind and body were crying out for oestrogen. We first tried natural oestrogen tablets, which helped the hot flushes but not her mental changes. Finally, much to the relief of Donna and her office staff, I prescribed a cream containing a combination of natural oestrogen and progesterone, which within a week produced a total relief of her mood swings and fatigue.

When it comes to treating pre-menstrual mood swings and loss of libido in older pre-menopausal women, my preference is to use natural oestrogen creams or patches rather than oestrogen tablets. The tablets must go through the liver and they induce the liver to make increased amounts of the protein called Sex Binding Hormone Globulin (SHBG). This SHBG binds (attaches to) the body's naturally produced progesterone and testosterone, which makes these hormones unavailable to the body, and this is why the tablet forms of hormones are often ineffective for the mood changes of the PMS. The hormone creams do not increase the production of SHBG and will produce blood levels of the natural hormones sufficient to suppress the cyclical hormonal highs and lows of the ovaries.

Can diuretics help PMS?

In women with severe pre-menstrual fluid retention and bloating, it may be necessary to use diuretic drugs. Some women find that they retain so much fluid that they gain up to five kilograms of weight during the seven days before menstrual bleeding. This is called cyclical oedema and may be extremely uncomfortable with a new wardrobe being required at this time of the month. In such cases, a special diuretic drug called a 'potassium sparing diuretic' such as Moduretic or Aldactone is excellent. These drugs remove unwanted fluid without causing a deficiency of the mineral potassium. Aldactone tablets in a dose of 25 to 100mg twice daily from day 14 to 28 of the menstrual cycle can help reduce fluid retention, acne and greasy skin. The use of raw juices made with a juice extracting machine and magnesium tablets such as Magnesium Complete will also help greatly with fluid retention.

Gonadotrophin Releasing Hormone Agonists (GnRH)

These are powerful synthetic hormones that act on the pituitary gland to completely inhibit the ovarian cycle. Their use results in a 'medical menopause' with very low levels of oestrogen and progesterone and absence of menstrual bleeding. They could only be recommended for severe PMS when all other hormonal and drug therapy has failed and then only on a short-term basis. Their long-term use would result in very low levels of oestrogen with increased risk of osteoporosis and cardiovascular disease.

Can antidepressant drugs help the PMS?

In women who do not respond to the use of natural hormone therapy the use of antidepressant drugs can bring relief from severe cyclical mood disorder that manifests pre-menstrually. Clinical trials have shown that the newer family of anti-depressant drugs known as Selective Serotonin Reuptake Inhibitors (SSRIs) are effective at relieving pre-menstrual depression and mood disorder (Ref 16,17). You may only need to take the medication during the 2 pre-menstrual weeks, or you may find that you need it every day, with an increase in the dosage during the 2 pre-menstrual weeks. Anti-depressant drugs are not habit forming and are very useful if there are a lot of outside stresses such as family issues, relationship problems, and low self esteem. Anti-depressants also help with sleep and anxiety if you suffer with insomnia. It is also wise to go to a professional counsellor to achieve more insight into how stress affects your behaviour and how to cope more efficiently with this.

We can help ourselves

I believe that the greatest healer is oneself. To heal ourselves, we need to be aware of certain helpful facts and guidelines. Firstly, the understanding that female sex hormone imbalance may play a role in depression is helpful. Women are more prone to depression than men, this depression usually starts after puberty, is worse pre-menstrually, after childbirth and during the zone of the peri-menopausal years. Without this understanding, these disturbances often continue with cyclical regularity and no one does anything effective about it, even though disorders like PMS and post natal depression are eminently treatable.

Women need to be aware of the biological model of psychological disorders where it is realised that our state of mind is influenced by our hormones, diet, nutritional status, drugs, lifestyle, exercise, general health and the environment, and not just by psychological factors.

If we can see womanhood as an advantage like a special gift, we are less likely to be intimidated by the cyclic nature of our biology, wanting to explore both its strengths and vulnerabilities. This is easier to enjoy when one knows that if the strengths diminish and the vulnerabilities increase, modern-day hormonal and nutritional therapy can restore the balance.

We need to tap into the wealth of healing resources and knowledge found in our inner selves to keep a balance with our accumulation of scientific and academic facts. By having faith in our inner female intuition, we can gain confidence in changing ourselves and any misguided situations around us. The skills of meditation and yoga can help us tune into the innate strength, peace and wisdom inside ourselves.

As an academic and eternal medical student, I have kept an open mind about new discoveries and this was partly the reason that I became interested in naturopathic medicine. It seemed to click with my inner sense of intuition and, no matter how much it was ridiculed or minimised by the establishment, it continued to make sense and produce good results. Like all doctors, I have accumulated considerable medical wisdom by communicating with my patients, who, together with my intuition, have both taught and inspired me for many years.

What are the Obstacles?

The attitude of some drug companies, doctors and psychiatrists is not always conducive to the active participation of women in their health dilemmas. Some doctors may prefer to keep control by fostering dependent relationships with their patients and keep them 'in the dark'. Other doctors may be reluctant to accept the biological causes of psychological disorders. There is an urgent need for more inter-specialty collaborative research to assess the role of hormones, nutritional supplements and drugs in various types of depression. Some psychiatrists (usually males) still see women through the teachings of Sigmund Freud, who believed that women were inherently more neurotic than men with their inability to resolve subconscious conflicts shown in the typical neuroses of depression, anxiety, hysteria or hypochondriasis. This narrow perspective leads to the stereotyping of women, reinforcing their inferiority and dependence upon mind-altering drugs.

In reality, today's woman is psychologically, if not hormonally, just as liberated and aware as today's man. She is increasingly reluctant to accept psychotropic drugs (especially sedatives, and tranquillisers) or synthetic hormones, in case they may take the edge off performance and blunt feelings and self expression.

It is interesting that sometimes it is not only psychiatrists, but also some feminists, who are cynical towards the idea that hormone fluctuations affect female psychology and behaviour. Such feminists also have a narrow perspective, preferring to say that the higher incidence of depression and suicide attempts in women is entirely due to environmental and psycho-social issues. They may feel it is demeaning or trivialising to admit that one's hormones could wreak mental havoc, fearing that this will give women a handicapping vulnerability or a uniquely female "Achilles heel". This attitude of denial is no longer appropriate and hormone therapy can enable us to compete and share with our male counterparts in a world where we need to keep our wits about us, not only for two, but for four weeks every month.

Another obstacle to overcome is the sometimes confused and conflicting messages about our hormones that are given to us by the media, lay press and 'pseudo experts', who have never had any clinical experience treating women with hormonal problems. We read negative and patronising articles with no clear strategies or hopes of cure offered. For example, we are told that PMS women should avoid giving dinner parties at that time of the month, as if the most serious implication was a collapsed soufflé or a lumpy sauce! This is ineffectual advice for the many professional women of today, who are surgeons, airline pilots or politicians. I was amazed when I read an article published in May 2004 in an American Aviation magazine, which was extremely derogatory to female professional pilots. Guess what? – The author was a male pilot! Basically he was saying that women pilots are easily spooked and don't have the physical strength, psychomotor co-ordination or steel nerves required to fly commercial airplanes. I was absolutely flabbergasted that this magazine had the gall to publish this article and I can just imagine the huge number of "letters to the editor" that this will provoke from their female readers. I would love to be "a fly on the wall" in their editor's office!

Another common obstacle is our self-image. Many women have very low self-esteem and are unable to love and admire themselves as unique individuals. They may find it uncomfortable to be assertive with their doctors or family. This lack of confidence makes it difficult for them to express their needs, anger, aggression or resentment when they really need to do this!

To overcome these limitations, the establishment of support groups for women with such problems as PMS, postnatal depression, drug dependence or midlife depression can be invaluable. Support groups provide an environment where women can begin to express themselves, building skills in confidence, creativity and self-assertiveness. For women who feel they have 'lost it', support groups can act as a stepping stone back into the real world.

Support groups can really open other avenues and take on many roles, such as sending a spokesperson for a radio interview, writing newspaper articles, inviting an expert speaker on women's health into your area, raising money for the local women's refuge, etc. They also provide psychological support for those women unable to afford counselling from a professional.

At the end of the day, we need to keep our sense of humour, which can be hard when the struggle for mental and physical harmony seems elusive, so the little cartoons in this chapter will help us laugh at ourselves. Yes, it's true now, as ever, laughter is a great form of medicine!

Helpful websites for emotional support and further information

www.npan.com.au

www.beyondblue.org.au

www.relationships.com.au

www.depression.com.au

www.anxietyaustralia.com.au

www.alcoholicsanonymous.org.au

www.moodgym.anu.edu.au

www.bluepages.anu.edu.au

www.crufad.unsw.edu.au

www.infrapsych.com

CHAPTER 3

Menstrual irregularity and absent menstruation

The duration of the menstrual cycle is calculated as the number of days between the first day of bleeding of your period to the first day of the next menstrual period. Not every woman has a cycle of exactly 28 days and the normal menstrual cycle can vary from 21 to 35 days.

It is not uncommon for the menstrual periods to become irregular and/or less frequent. If a woman, who previously had regular monthly cycles, fails to menstruate for over three months, she has what doctors call amenorrhoea and this is not a normal state in a non-pregnant premenopausal women. So basically the absence of menstruation in a woman who is not menopausal or pregnant is called amenorrhoea.

What are the causes of infrequent or irregular menstruation?

In the vast majority of cases, a hormonal imbalance resulting in failure to ovulate is the cause of irregular or infrequent menstruation. Hormonal imbalances disturb the menstrual clock in the hypothalamus and the sensitive communication link between the hypothalamus, pituitary gland and ovaries. (see Diagram 4, page 16).

Disorders of the uterus and/or a possible blockage of the cervix or vagina can also result in absent menstruation.

Let us take a look at some of the more common causes of absent or irregular menstrual cycles-

1. Changes in body weight

The menstrual clock can be switched off by rapid or marked changes in body weight with either weight loss or weight gain having this effect.

Body fat produces both female and male sex hormones and so very thin women have lower levels of these hormones in their bodies. In addition, if the menstrual clock has switched off as a protective mechanism against extreme thinness, ovulation will not occur and thus the ovaries will produce very little sex hormones. These very low levels of sex hormones can cause menstrual bleeding to cease. If weight can be gained back to achieve a normal body weight relative to body height, the menstrual clock should restart causing a resumption of regular menstrual bleeding. Women who suffer with eating disorders such as anorexia or bulimia may find that their rapid and marked changes in body weight cause the menstrual cycle to become disrupted. In women who are dependent on drugs such as narcotics or amphetamines the body weight may fluctuate greatly producing an irregular menstrual cycle.

In underweight women prolonged periods of amenorrhoea are usually associated with very low oestrogen levels, which may cause premature bone loss resulting in osteoporosis. A bone density test should be done in such cases to check for bone thinning.

Overweight women tend to produce some oestrogen and excess levels of male hormones (androgens) from their fat tissue and ovaries but do not produce adequate amounts of progesterone. They often have poly-cystic ovaries (see page 153), which do not ovulate regularly and pro-duce oestrogen and plenty of androgens but insufficient progesterone. They fail to menstruate regularly because their uterus is exposed to oestrogen without the progesterone required to induce a withdrawal bleed. Once again, the achievement of a normal body weight relative to body height (normal Body Mass Index) will usually bring back regular ovulation and regular menstrual cycles and more balanced levels of the female and male sex hormones.

For more information on Body Mass Index and the latest weight loss strategies, see my book titled "*Can't Lose Weight? You could have Syndrome X*"

HEIGHT FOR WEIGHT GRAPH

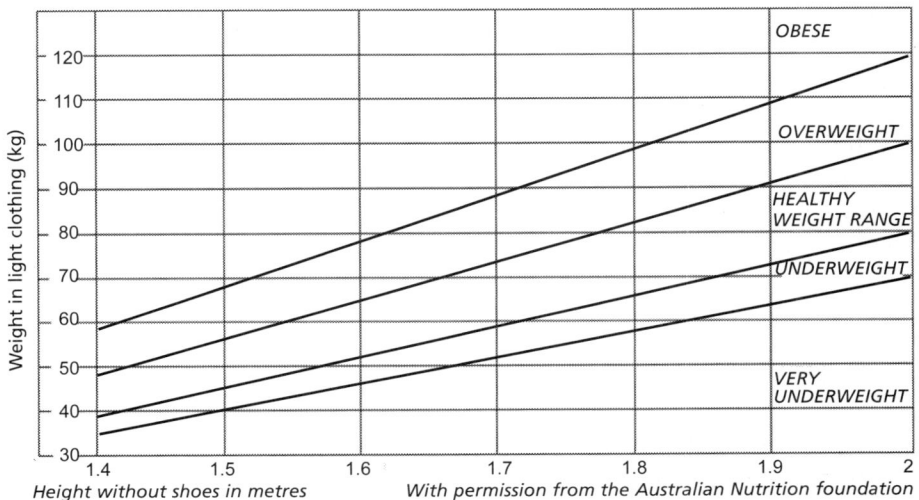

Height without shoes in metres　　With permission from the Australian Nutrition foundation

2. Imbalances in Exercise

Excessive exercise can switch off the menstrual clock resulting in amenorrhoea. These women may be athletes or very sportive and are often muscular with low amounts of body fat and thus low levels of sex hormones. High levels of exercise are more likely to cause amenorrhoea if the diet is deficient in healthy fats, proteins and carbohydrates, so it is important to have your diet assessed by a professional. If the amenorrhoea persists, they will be at a higher risk of osteoporosis despite their vigorous physical workouts.

3. Stress

Stress and emotional trauma can act on the hypothalamus to switch off the menstrual clock and in such cases, menstruation may not resume until a woman is feeling happy and relaxed. Some women lose their menstrual periods after a traumatic relationship or divorce and find that their periods return when they fall in love again.

4. Imbalances of the Pituitary Gland

The pituitary gland produces several hormones that have an effect on the function of the ovaries and thus the menstrual cycle. These hormones are Follicle Stimulating Hormone (FSH), Luteinising Hormone (LH), Thyroid Stimulating Hormone (TSH) and Prolactin, and these hormones can all be measured accurately with a simple blood test. If the pituitary gland produces excessive amounts of the lactation hormone prolactin this may lead to amenorrhoea. This is because the high levels of prolactin switch off the menstrual clock and the ovaries, which is why it is normal for breast feeding mothers to miss their periods while they are breast feeding regularly. If a non-lactating woman has excessive prolactin production from the pituitary gland, she may stop menstruating, which is not a normal situation. The high levels of prolactin may cause the secretion of breast milk from the nipple, which is called inappropriate lactation. If the blood levels of prolactin are significantly elevated (more than four times the upper limit of normal) an investigation of the pituitary gland for the presence of a prolactin-secreting tumour must be done. If the prolactin level is only slightly elevated it can usually be brought down over a period of several months by a change in diet and lifestyle, and if needed, the medication called bromocriptine. For blood levels of prolactin - see page 177.

Excessive prolactin production may result from

■ Some types of medications such as anti-depressants
■ Severe stress

- Unexplained hormonal imbalances in the hypothalamus
- A small tumour in the pituitary gland that secretes prolactin.
  This tumour is usually a benign (non-cancerous) adenoma growing within the pituitary gland, and it may be very small in size when it is known as a micro-adenoma. These tumours are found with an MRI (Magnetic Resonance Imaging) scan or CAT (computerized axial tomography) scan of the pituitary gland.

Treatment of elevated prolactin

The drug bromocriptine (Parlodel) can reduce prolactin levels and usually restores regular menstruation and fertility. Parlodel is taken orally everyday and is started in a small dose to avoid its common side effect of nausea. The dose of the Parlodel is gradually increased until the prolactin level has returned to normal. It is practical to take the Parlodel with the evening meal so that nausea occurs while sleeping. The other drug that can be used to lower prolactin is called Cabergoline and it is given twice a week only.

In some patients even after prolactin levels are suppressed back to normal levels, ovulation will not resume and menstruation remains absent. Often in such cases success can be achieved with an improvement in diet and lifestyle and nutritional supplementation.

In my own clinical practice I have found that women with elevated levels of prolactin will often respond to a change in diet with the elimination of ALL dairy products. For some as yet unexplained reason the hormones found in cow's milk and its products (cheese, butter, cream, yogurt, ice-cream etc) overstimulate the pituitary gland causing it to manufacture excess amounts of prolactin. I have seen dramatic reductions in the blood levels of prolactin after the patient has completely eliminated all dairy products from her diet. It is also important to ensure that your diet is high in antioxidants, which are best obtained from fruits, vegetables and raw juices. A supplement of selenium (containing selenomethionine) to provide a daily dose of 100 to 200mcg can help to shrink benign pituitary tumours.

For more information call the Health Advisory Service on 0246558855.

Empty sella syndrome

Another problem that can affect the pituitary gland is that of "empty sella syndrome". The pituitary gland is situated at the base of the brain and is surrounded and protected by a bony part of the skull called the sella turcica (meaning Turkish saddle). If a CAT or MRI scan of the sella turcica cannot detect the pituitary gland within it, the sella is obviously empty and the patient is diagnosed with "empty sella syndrome". These brain imaging techniques of CT or MRI will show that the sella is enlarged and the pituitary gland cannot be seen or is very small.

There are 2 types of empty sella syndrome

Primary empty sella syndrome

In most cases the function of the pituitary gland is normal and there are no serious symptoms. In around 10% to 15% of these patients the level of prolactin may be elevated, which leads to absent menstruation (amenorrhoea). Elevated fluid pressure may occur inside the skull in around 10% of patients and this may produce headaches. Another relatively common symptom is a runny nose (rhinorrhoea). Some patients may complain of low libido and sexual dysfunction.

It is more common in women who are overweight or who have high blood pressure.

Primary empty sella syndrome is caused by an increase in pressure inside the space in the sella turcica, and this squashes the pituitary gland so that it becomes flattened out along the bony walls of the sella. In some cases there may be a chronic inflammatory problem in the area of the sella, which is increasing the pressure and this can be improved with high dose antioxidants obtained from juicing of raw vegetables and a complete antioxidant formula containing selenium.

Primary empty sella syndrome is not a serious health problem and does not reduce life span.

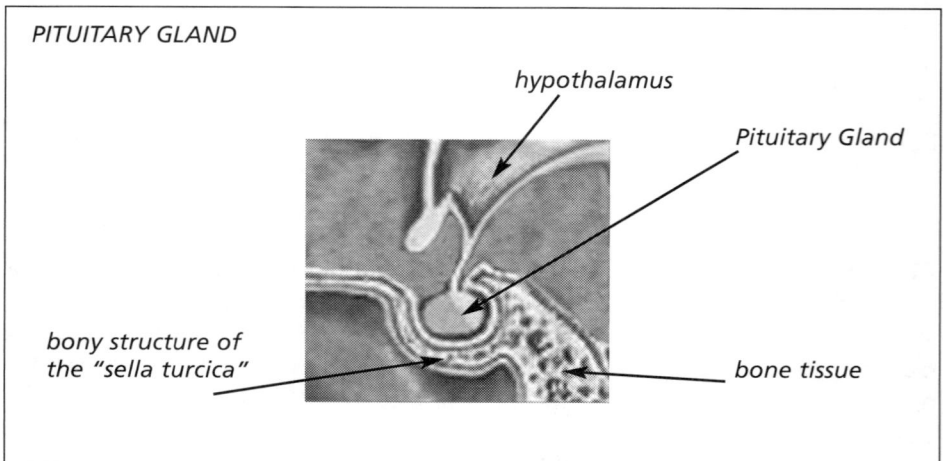

PITUITARY GLAND

hypothalamus

Pituitary Gland

bony structure of
the "sella turcica"

bone tissue

Secondary empty sella syndrome

In these cases the sella becomes empty because of another reason such as a pituitary tumour, brain haemorrhage (stroke), head injury, surgery or radiation therapy to the area of the pituitary gland. In these cases the pituitary gland is often damaged and does not produce adequate amounts of all or some of its hormones – this condition of pituitary gland underactivity is called hypopituitarism. Therapy is designed to replace the hormones that are deficient as a result of the pituitary gland underactivity.

In children and adolescents the empty sella syndrome is often associated with abnormal production of hormones from the pituitary gland such as a deficiency of growth hormone.

For more information on disorders of the pituitary gland including the empty sella syndrome visit www.umm.edu/endocrin/sella.htm

5. Imbalances in the function of the thyroid gland

Thyroid dysfunction can result in menstrual irregularity or amenorrhoea and this can occur if the thyroid gland is overactive or underactive. When the thyroid imbalance is corrected, regular menstrual bleeding and fertility will resume.

For more information on the thyroid gland see page 130

6. Premature Menopause

Premature menopause is defined as ovarian failure occurring under the age of forty years. When this occurs menstrual bleeding will become less and less frequent and eventually stop altogether.

Spontaneous premature menopause occurs in approximately 1% of women. There is an increased incidence of up to 10% of premature menopause, after gynaecological surgery, chemotherapy and radiotherapy for cancer.

For more information on premature menopause see page 51.

The treatment of amenorrhoea

The treatment of the amenorrhoea varies depending upon the cause.

If a premenopausal woman with absent menstruation is sexually active and does not want to become pregnant, a suitable treatment is the Oral Contraceptive Pill (OCP). This will restore regular menstruation and protect the bones from osteoporosis in the underweight woman with low oestrogen levels.

In overweight women with high or normal oestrogen levels, natural progesterone, synthetic progesterone or the OCP will restore a regular menstrual bleed and protect the uterus from cancer. Generally speaking natural progesterone is the preferred choice, as it does not cause side effects such as weight gain, depression or problems with cholesterol. Natural progesterone will not provide any contraception.

Polycystic Ovarian Syndrome (PCOS) can cause amenorrhoea associated with excessive levels of male hormones resulting in acne, facial hair and weight excess. The OCP can reduce excessive levels of male hormones and produce a regular menstrual bleed in these women and suitable brands of the OCP are Diane and Yasmin. If contraception is not required, natural progesterone or the anti-male progestogen known as cyproterone acetate (Androcur) can produce a regular menstrual bleed, as well as help to relieve the other symptoms of PCOS.

If the amenorrhoea is associated with persistent infertility, it is necessary to stimulate ovulation with fertility drugs, such as clomiphene or gonadotrophin drugs. These drugs should be given by a specialist gynaecologist.

NORMAL OVARIAN CYCLE

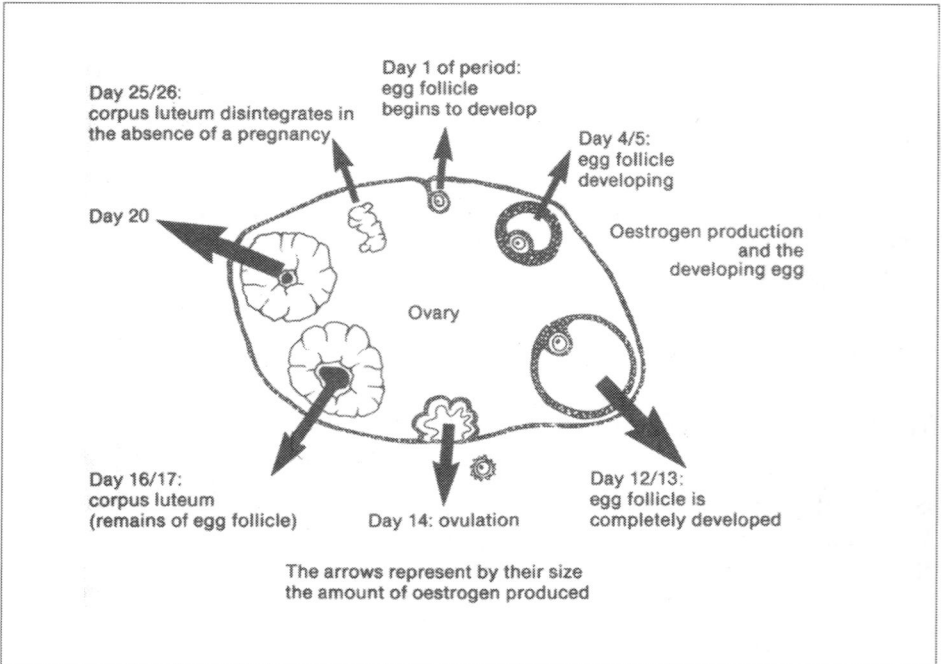

Day 25/26:
corpus luteum disintegrates in the absence of a pregnancy

Day 1 of period:
egg follicle begins to develop

Day 4/5:
egg follicle developing

Day 20

Oestrogen production and the developing egg

Ovary

Day 16/17:
corpus luteum (remains of egg follicle)

Day 14: ovulation

Day 12/13:
egg follicle is completely developed

The arrows represent by their size the amount of oestrogen produced

Premature Menopause

Premature menopause is defined as ovarian failure occurring under the age of forty years. Spontaneous premature menopause occurs in approximately 1% of women.

What are the causes of premature menopause?

- In many cases the cause is unknown, and is due to spontaneous premature ovarian failure
- Auto-immune diseases – these may be associated with multiple gland failures, such as thyroid and adrenal gland dysfunction, as well as ovarian failure
- Heavy smoking may damage the blood supply to the ovaries
- Genetic factors – X chromosome deletions, or rare karyotypes such as 47XXX
- After gynaecological surgery – such as hysterectomy or removal of the ovaries
- Chemotherapy and/or radiotherapy for cancer

How do we diagnose premature menopause?

1. There must be at least four months of absent menstrual bleeding
2. There must be elevated blood levels of the pituitary gland hormone called Follicle Stimulating Hormone (FSH), on 2 separate occasions, with the blood being tested for FSH levels at least 6 weeks apart. To qualify for menopause the FSH levels should be over 40mU/mL

Other tests, which may be done, are
- Oestrogen and progesterone blood levels, which would be low
- A trans-vaginal ultrasound scan to look for the existence of ovarian eggs (follicles), which will be absent or shrunken if the ovaries have failed
- Chromosomal testing to check for genetic causes

What are the symptoms of premature menopause?

The symptoms of premature menopause vary quite a lot depending upon if the failure of the ovaries occurs gradually, or very suddenly. This is why blood tests for FSH levels are so important, as they provide the definitive diagnosis.

Possible presenting symptoms of premature menopause are

- Absent menstruation
- Loss of fertility
- Irregular and/or infrequent periods
- Very light or heavy periods
- Mood disorders
- Loss of libido
- Vaginal dryness & discomfort during sex
- Aches and pains
- Night sweats and/or poor sleep
- Fatigue

After surgical removal of the ovaries, or destruction of the ovaries by radio-therapy or chemotherapy, the onset of menopausal symptoms is usually sudden and often quite dramatic, especially in younger women.

Problems associated with premature menopause are

- Increased rate of bone loss
- Possible increased risk of cardiovascular disease
- Possible psychological, sexual and emotional problems
- Premature loss of fertility – although in a significant percentage of women with premature ovarian failure, the ovaries may temporarily come back to life, and in around 10% of cases, a spontaneous pregnancy may subsequently occur. In women with true premature ovarian failure, we usually cannot get the ovaries to produce eggs, which will ovulate. If these women wish to have children, they will need to consider adoption or receiving an ovarian egg from a donor.

Psychological issues of Premature Menopause

It is not uncommon for women with premature menopause, to experience a range of negative feelings such as

Shock & disbelief
A sense of great loss
A sense of isolation from women of their own age group
A sense of being cheated, especially if fertility is desired
A sense of being different or abnormal
A fear of premature ageing
A fear of loss of sexuality

It is very important that after the diagnosis is made, a woman has ample time and opportunity to express her emotions. Her partner should also be present for some discussion of the meaning of premature menopause.

Some women erroneously believe that they have a disease, or that their relationships will never be the same; thus a lot of reassurance and positive feedback is required. The term "premature menopause" may conjure up negative connotations of being old, undesirable, barren or inadequate, and it is more acceptable to the patient and her partner, family and friends to use the expression of "premature ovarian failure."

Helpful web sites are www.whas.com.au and www.pofsupport.org

Treatment of premature menopause

The risk of osteoporosis is greater in women, who have a premature menopause, and in the past, relatively high dose combined oral HRT, or oral contraceptive pills have usually been prescribed.

This has been done to relieve symptoms of oestrogen deficiency, and to preserve bone density. Indeed many women are given the oral contraceptive pill, as this induces a regular period, so that women will know they are not pregnant. This is comforting to women who feel that the 10% spontaneous pregnancy rate after premature ovarian failure is unacceptable.

There are many types of HRT that can be prescribed and generally a dose of oestrogen that is equivalent to 0.625mg of Premarin, or the 100mcg oestrogen patches is used. To produce a regular period (withdrawal bleed), a synthetic progestogen such as Provera, is given for 12 to 14 days of each month. Alternately micronised natural progesterone capsules in a dose of 100 to 200mg daily can be used instead of synthetic progesterone. This type of treatment will help with symptoms of oestrogen deficiency, and may help well-being and sex drive; however some women will also need testosterone. Testosterone can be given in the form of a cream, gel or lozenge.

If the premature menopause was due to surgical removal of the uterus and/or ovaries, then many women find that implants of oestrogen and testosterone, provide a complete relief of symptoms, and greatly enhance the sex life. Natural progesterone can be given to balance these hormones; however it is not available in implants so creams or troches will need to be prescribed.

The new-generation synthetic HRT called Livial (Tibolone) can provide a welcome relief of symptoms, and also maintain bone density. Theoretically Livial should be less likely to increase the incidence of breast cancer than conventional combined oral HRT, because Livial exerts an anti-oestrogenic effect upon the breast. I have had several patients who are taking Livial, who have told me that it has made a big improvement in the quality of their life. Other patients have told me that they have tried Livial, and found that it made them feel "bland" and caused weight gain. Once again this shows me that every woman's response to HRT is very individual.

In the light of the Women's Health Initiative study (WHI), which showed that long term combined HRT using oral oestrogens and synthetic progestogens, will increase the incidence of breast cancer and blood clots, a significant percentage of women with premature menopause, will not feel comfortable about taking these tablets. Thankfully we now have safer alternatives available for long term HRT, such as hormone patches and creams; some women will also be candidates for oral natural oestrogens and natural progesterone.

Transdermal types of oestrogen (patches or creams) can be combined with a natural or synthetic progesterone, and natural testosterone if needed. For a woman who loses her sex hormones under the age of 40, the prospect of a life without any sex hormones in her body, can be daunting. She will probably live another 40 years, and without sex hormones, she may feel totally sexless, tired, and unfeminine.

The use of natural therapies and mineral supplements can help greatly in the relief of symptoms and the maintenance of bone density; however when it comes to sexuality and sensuality, these natural therapies cannot replace the effect of real hormones. Thus most women with premature ovarian failure will want to try a combination of natural therapies and some form of HRT.

Case History

Jenny provides an interesting case history for younger women going through a premature ovarian failure. Jenny had undergone a hysterectomy when she was 38 years old, for severe endometriosis. Her disease had been so wide-spread, that the surgeon had not been able to conserve her ovaries. Thus she had woken up from the operation with no uterus and no ovaries. Within 4 days of the operation, she had symptoms of severe hormone deficiency, and her hot flushes were so frequent that she was unable to sleep. Her gynaecologist had prescribed Trisequens tablets to be taken continuously, and these worked reasonably well for 6 months. Trisequens contains a combination of natural oestrogen and synthetic progesterone in one tablet. Jenny had decided to see me because she had found that the hormone tablets she was taking had caused her to gain 12 kilograms in weight and had made her feel bloated. She also complained that although she was now free of pelvic pain, she did not feel particularly feminine, and had no sex drive. Jenny had read about natural

HRT, and wondered if it might suit her better. Jenny's blood tests showed that she had reasonable levels of oestradiol, but very low levels of natural progesterone, and a very low free androgen index (FAI). This meant that although she was receiving enough oestrogen, she was very deficient in natural progesterone and male hormones. The oral hormones that she was taking were making her liver produce excessive amounts of the hormone-binding protein called Sex Hormone Binding Globulin (SHBG). Her high levels of SHBG were binding the majority of the hormones in her blood stream, which meant that her hormones were being inactivated. I explained to Jenny that we needed to do several things to re-balance her hormones –

1. Reduce her high levels of SHBG, which would free up her active hormones
2. Increase her blood levels of natural progesterone
3. Increase her blood levels of natural testosterone
4. Maintain her blood oestrogen levels

To achieve these changes I recommended the following –

1. That she stop the oral hormones, which could have been causing weight gain and bloating. The oral hormones were also increasing her SHBG levels.
2. That she begin a troche containing a combination of Tri-est 2mg, natural progesterone 40mg, and natural testosterone 1mg daily, which she would place between the upper gum and the cheek, until it slowly absorbed through the cheek, into the circulation.
3. That she begin a hormone cream containing a mixture of oestradiol 1mg, natural progesterone 20mg, and natural testosterone 1mg, which she would massage into the vulva and clitoral area every night.
4. That she start a raw juicing program and take a liver tonic to promote weight loss and reduce fluid retention.

I asked her to return to see me after 4 months of using this program, at which stage I would retest her hormone levels. After 4 months on this program, Jenny's blood results showed that her hormones were now in the correct balance; her progesterone levels were now in the normal range, and her SHBG had reduced considerably and her FAI was back to normal levels. Jenny told me, that she was not surprised, that her blood tests showed her hormones were back in balance. She had lost 8 kilograms and felt happy with her appearance. She was particularly happy about the improvement in her sex life; now she was free of pain, and her hormones were back in balance, her sex life had not been better in many years, she said. She felt much happier about the prospect of taking natural hormones long term, than she had felt about taking synthetic progestogen.

CHAPTER 5

Gynaecological problems associated with hormonal imbalances

Endometriosis

This is a common disorder affecting around 10% of premenopausal women. In this disorder the lining of the uterus (endometrium) grows backwards through the uterine tubes (fallopian tubes) and spills out the ends of the tubes into the pelvic and abdominal cavities. Once inside these cavities it implants upon various organs such as the bladder, the ovaries, the bowel and the outside of the uterus where it starts to grow like a weed. The weed-like endometrial implants are influenced by the female sex hormones oestrogen and progesterone; oestrogen makes them grow while progesterone makes them bleed. These endometrial deposits grow and bleed each month causing bleeding inside the pelvic and abdominal cavities from where there is no escape to the outside. This abnormal internal bleeding can result in cysts, blood clots and scar tissue (adhesions) on the bowel, the bladder, the ovaries and the outside of the uterus and fallopian tubes. This results in abdominal and pelvic pain during menstrual bleeding and also at other times during the menstrual cycle. Low back ache may also occur if the endometrial implants grow in the small pouch behind the uterus which is adjacent to the lower bowel.

Other symptoms that may be caused by endometriosis are
- Abdominal bloating and swelling
- Constipation or diarrhoea
- Bladder problems
- Painful sexual intercourse
- Heavy painful periods
- Anaemia, iron deficiency and fatigue
- Ovulation pain at mid-cycle
- Bleeding or spotting between menstrual bleeding
- Infertility due to blockage of the tubes and damage to the ovaries

Endometriosis is the most common cause of chronic pain in women in the reproductive age group and is found in over 20% of infertile women.

What causes endometriosis?

Genetic factors – there is often a family history of endometriosis.

Poor immune function – this prevents the immune cells from destroying the abnormally sited endometrial tissue and allows excess inflammation to occur.

Dietary factors – if your diet is high in saturated fat, dairy products and refined carbohydrates you will find that endometriosis is more likely to occur. Deficiencies of anti-oxidants and minerals can also weaken the immune system.

Hormonal imbalances – characterised by a relative deficiency of progesterone compared to body oestrogen levels.

How is endometriosis diagnosed?

If you suspect that you have endometriosis you should see a specialist gynaecologist who will do a thorough general and pelvic examination. The gynaecologist will perform key-hole surgery in the form of a laparoscopy. During this procedure the doctor can look directly into the abdominal and pelvic cavities through an operating telescope (laparoscope) passed through a tiny incision in the abdominal wall. Of course you will be under a general anaesthetic. Laparoscopy is the most accurate way to diagnose endometriosis especially in its early and curable stages.

It is important that you seek a prompt referral to a specialist gynaecologist, as it is not uncommon for the correct diagnosis to be delayed. Some women with endometriosis are incorrectly told that they have irritable bowel syndrome, normal period pains, pelvic inflammatory disease or a psychosomatic illness!

Treatment options for endometriosis

Drug therapy

The drugs used to treat this disease act by shrinking the abnormal endometrial deposits and cysts and preventing new deposits from forming. They do this by blocking the production and/or effects of oestrogen. These drugs can be used as an alternative to surgery in mild cases, as an addition to surgery in more severe cases, preventative therapy before IVF, and before surgery to shrink the endometrial deposits and make the surgery easier.

The drugs that may be used include

Danazol

Danazol is an "anti-oestrogen" which blocks the effects of oestrogen in your body and thus shrinks the endometrial deposits. Danazol has male hormone like effects and its side effects may include weight gain, acne, facial hair and hot flushes.

Gonadotrophin – releasing hormone analogues

An example of these drugs is nafarelin (Synarel). These drugs stop the ovaries from producing sex hormones by putting your body into a temporary menopause. They may produce an initial flare up of the endometriosis, but eventually will control the disease. They will cause menopause like symptoms as a side effect. Prolonged use of these drugs causes a loss of bone density and they cannot be taken for more than 6 months at a time. They are taken as a nasal spray.

You should avoid pregnancy while taking these drugs and although they are often dramatically effective, still around 10% of women will not be helped by them. Drug therapy shrinks the endometrial deposits but they may not disappear completely and recurrence of endometriosis within one year of stopping these drugs is common.

Progesterone

If the endometriosis is severe it will probably be necessary to use the stronger synthetic progestogens at least initially. Examples of the synthetic progestogens are Provera and Primolut and quite large doses may be required initially; they are taken every day of the menstrual cycle.

Once the symptoms become less severe, natural progesterone can be used and most women prefer this, as it does not cause the unpleasant side effects that the synthetic progestogens may cause in some women. The dose of natural progesterone required may be quite high, at least initially, with 400mg daily being prescribed. Once the balancing effect has kicked in, the dose of natural progesterone can be reduced way down to a maintenance dose. The maintenance dose will vary from 35 to 200mg daily. The natural progesterone can be given in the form of troches (lozenges), capsules or a cream. The cream can be rubbed into the skin or inserted high up into the vagina last thing at night on retiring. It is quite safe to stay on long term natural progesterone to control endometriosis. Many women find that natural progesterone is a very effective and safe long term method of controlling endometriosis.

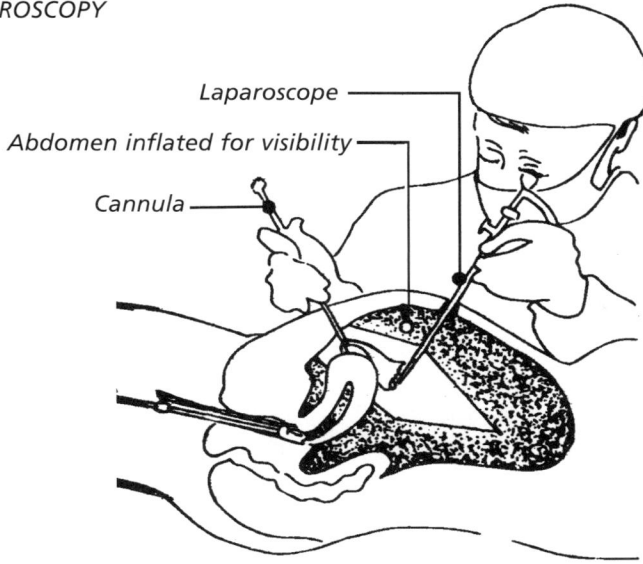

LAPAROSCOPY

Laparoscope

Abdomen inflated for visibility

Cannula

Endometriosis is like a weed and thus tends to grow back or recur, and this is why it is important to combine any drug or hormonal therapy with nutritional medicine. This will greatly reduce the recurrence rates and enable you to avoid repetitive surgery with its attendant complications of scar tissue, intestinal obstruction and chronic pain.

Surgery

Generally this can be done via key-hole surgery through a laparoscope and major abdominal surgery can be avoided. The surgeon can remove the endometrial implants using laser surgery and thus is able to target the abnormal tissue more accurately. Unfortunately around one third of patients will get a recurrence of the endometriosis after surgery and will require repeated laparoscopies. If you get a recurrence it is advisable to consult a specialist in advanced laparoscopic surgery. Severe recurrent endometriosis may be extensive and require removal of one or both ovaries, the uterus or even part of the bladder or bowel. When medical therapy and conservative surgery have failed to cure the endometriosis and chronic pain is an everyday reality, the uterus and ovaries often need to be removed. Hormone replacement therapy is not given for 3 months after hysterectomy and removal of the ovaries to allow any hidden endometriosis to shrink first.

The earlier that nutritional medicine is begun the better your chances of a cure of this painful disease will be. This type of treatment is aimed at strengthening the immune system and reducing inflammation with a gradual disappearance of the endometrial implants being achieved.

The recommended program consists of

- Boosting the intake of antioxidants by raw juicing and taking a supplement containing selenium, zinc, and vitamin E and vitamin C. Selenium Complete tablets contain these ingredients and the dose is 3 tablets daily. Raw juicing is vital and suitable things to juice are raw red and green apples, citrus fruits, purple cabbage, beetroot, capsicums, spinach, pineapple, ginger root and carrot. If you can juice everyday your chances of success will be higher.

- The powder called MSM (Methyl Sulphonyl Methane) combined with vitamin C can be very helpful because it provides organic sulphur, which helps to reduce adhesions and helps the liver to detoxify excessive oestrogen.

- Increasing your intake of legumes (beans, lentils & chickpeas), raw nuts and seeds.

- Increasing your intake of essential fatty acids from cold pressed oils such as flaxseed oil, olive oil, grape seed oil and oily fish.

- Increasing your intake of fibre from whole grains, raw nuts and seeds and raw fruits and vegetable salads.

- Some women find that they are much better if they avoid all dairy products, presumably because cow's milk products produce unfavourable hormonal influences upon endometriosis. You can substitute cow's milk with soy milk, rice milk, almond milk, oat milk or coconut milk.

- If possible eat organic free range poultry and eggs.

- Avoid deep fried foods and processed foods containing white flour, hydrogenated oils and refined sugars.

- A regular exercise program is important and some women find that yoga is excellent in reducing pain and pelvic congestion.

- Make sure that you are well hydrated by drinking at least 2 litres of water daily.

Even if you have had surgery and/or require strong drugs, the use of nutritional medicine is extremely valuable, as it is treating the cause of endometriosis and is going to provide you with the greatest chance of cure. Nutritional medicine does not work over night and you need to be regular, disciplined and persistent, as you may not see results for several months. It is truly worth the effort and I have had many success stories in my patients who have achieved a complete remission of their disease after 6 months.

Heavy painful periods

The problem of excess blood loss during menstrual bleeding is called menorrhagia and this is usually defined as heavy blood loss that cannot be absorbed by a menstrual pad and is often associated with the passage of large blood clots. If the heavy bleeding continues for more than 6 days iron deficiency anaemia becomes likely. This type of anaemia will cause severe fatigue and possible dizziness.

Menorrhagia can be associated with an enlarged or fibroid uterus, polyps in the uterus or pelvic infection. It may also be caused by bleeding and clotting disorders of the blood that need to be checked for with special blood tests. If these disorders are excluded and no underlying cause for the heavy bleeding can be found and the heavy bleeding persists, this type of bleeding is called "dysfunctional uterine bleeding". In the vast majority of cases dysfunctional uterine bleeding is caused by the hormonal imbalance called "oestrogen dominance" where there is a relative deficiency of progesterone production from the ovaries.

Women with heavy, irregular and/or painful periods should consult a specialist gynaecologist who will insert a telescope through the vagina into the uterus to have a good look at the uterine cavity. This telescope is called a hysteroscope and the doctor can take samples of the uterine lining or perform surgery to the uterus through the hysteroscope. In all women with very heavy and/or irregular bleeding a proper and full investigation must be done by a specialist gynaecologist to exclude endometrial cancer (cancer of the uterus) which is not uncommon. One can never be too careful and unfortunately uterine cancer is still missed often enough today, because women and doctors assume that heavy and/or irregular bleeding must be hormonal in origin.

If the heavy bleeding persists the lining of the uterus can be removed via the hysteroscope and this procedure is called endometrial ablation. Ablation often produces an excellent result with a dramatic reduction or even cessation of menstrual bleeding. Ablation of the endometrium will not always improve menstrual pain, and indeed may cause menstrual pain to worsen. For this reason it is always wise to try more natural therapies first.

In the majority of women the oral contraceptive pill will control heavy and/or painful periods very well, however if contraception is not required, these problems can be controlled with either synthetic or natural progesterone. Natural progesterone is usually more popular with women because it is most unlikely to cause any side effects and usually reduces the heavy bleeding effectively. Doses of natural progesterone of 100 to 400mg daily are usually effective in controlling painful and/or heavy menstrual bleeding. Natural progesterone can be given in the form of troches, capsules or creams. The cream can be rubbed into the skin or the cream can be inserted high up into the vagina last thing at night on retiring to bed.

Antioxidants are important and often reduce the amount of bleeding and vitamin C is the most important, with doses of 2000 to 4000mg daily being required. Vitamin K is able to reduce heavy bleeding and the best sources of vitamin K are oily fish and green leafy vegetables. The regular juicing of raw carrots, spinach, kale, green string beans, wheat grass, apple, citrus and beetroot can produce a huge reduction in the amount of menstrual blood loss and pain.

Essential fatty acids are able to reduce the production of pain-producing inflammatory chemicals and I recommend that you supplement your diet with cold pressed flaxseed oil and fish oil. If this is insufficient you may have to resort to anti-prostaglandin drugs such as Ponstan or Naprogesic when the period pain is anticipated.

CHAPTER 6

Hormonal Headaches

During my practice of medicine, I have seen countless women, who complain that around the time of menstrual bleeding, they are plagued with horrible headaches. These headaches may occur during the several days preceding the onset of the menstrual blood flow or during menstruation. They can also occur around mid-cycle at the time of ovulation. We call these repetitive cyclical headaches "hormonal" in type, as during these times, the blood levels of the sex hormones undergo rapid or large changes. (see Diagram 7, page 64)

Every woman suffering with regular headaches should keep a menstrual and headache calendar to illustrate a possible hormonal link. If hormones are the trigger factor for the headaches, a six-month calendar record will demonstrate the headache pattern. (See Maria's Calendar Page 66).

The hormonal pattern of these headaches can change as a woman gets older, after childbirth, after hysterectomy or after surgical sterilisation when the tubes are tied (tubal ligation). These factors may be associated with an overall decrease in the production of oestrogen and/or progesterone from the ovaries, when the usual cyclical drop in blood hormones becomes more extreme, causing the headaches to be more frequent, more severe and to last longer.

One woman, aged 40, who came to see me complained of anxiety and depression and a migraine headache every second day. She said she'd been like this for ten years ever since the removal of her uterus and one ovary at the age of 30. Yes, you guessed it, she had never received any Hormone Replacement Therapy (HRT). Thankfully, she had the common sense to avoid taking painkillers for her chronic headaches or she may very well have needed dialysis for analgesic induced kidney disease. She had resorted to taking ergotamine tablets every day to constrict the throbbing swollen blood vessels in her head, but this made her nauseated and caused her hands and feet to be blue and cold. She felt sexless, miserable and trapped in the body of a woman older than her years. Her blood tests revealed extremely low levels of oestrogen and progesterone.

After receiving natural oestrogen in the form of an implant, she blossomed in a matter of four weeks into a serene and happy woman and I discovered that she had a delightful personality buried under all that pain. Her headaches became a rare event and she coped better with her family stresses than ever before. Once the implant wore off, I planned to maintain her on a cream containing natural oestrogen and progesterone.

There were several reasons why she had taken so long to find relief. Firstly, her doctor had not recognised that migraine is often exacerbated by hormonal imbalances and secondly, after she had been told that, "you have to learn to live with it", she felt guilty about complaining to doctors and was not sufficiently assertive in her pursuit of relief.

Why do hormonal imbalances cause headaches?

The reason why imbalances in blood oestrogen and/or progesterone levels may cause our head to ache is not fully understood. These sex hormones are steroid hormones and, as such, probably exert an anti-inflammatory effect upon the musculoskeletal tissues, and a stabilising effect upon the blood vessels. It is logical that when blood levels of these hormones fluctuate, this could trigger off an inflammatory and destabilising effect upon the blood vessels in the head. This is experienced as a throbbing pain, as the blood vessels constrict and then dilate excessively. We call this a 'vascular headache,' and if the disturbance to the brain's circulation is severe, a typical migraine headache may develop.

Someone who suffers with regular migraines is known as a 'migraineur'. True migraine may be associated with visual disturbances such as temporary loss of vision and bright flashing lights and vomiting, and may last for

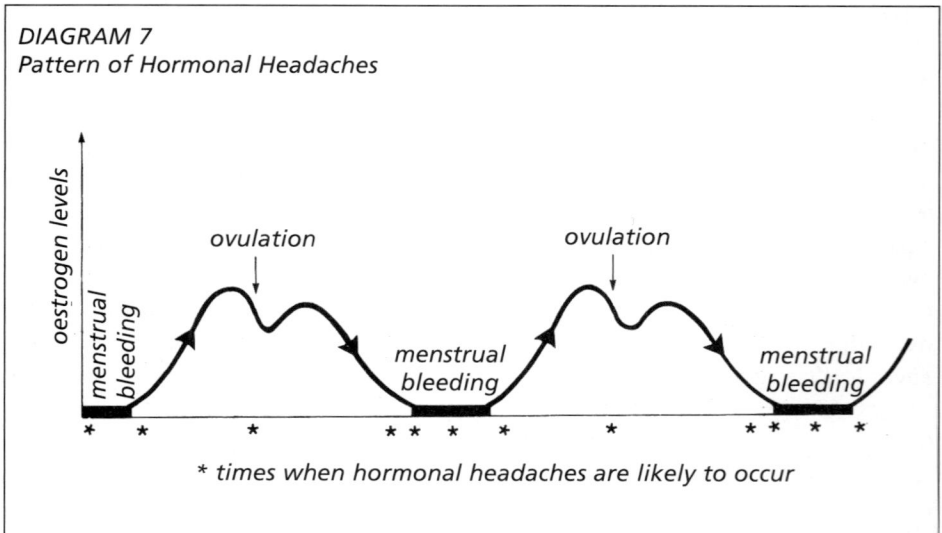

DIAGRAM 7
Pattern of Hormonal Headaches

oestrogen levels

menstrual bleeding

ovulation

ovulation

menstrual bleeding

menstrual bleeding

* times when hormonal headaches are likely to occur

24 to 48 hours unless treatment is given. Women with hormonal headaches will often complain that the bones and muscles in their head and face are aching and tender to touch, and in these cases, a therapeutic massage on the tender trigger points can be helpful. Hormonal headaches may be associated with general body aches and pains, fatigue and depression, which reflects the low levels of oestrogen and/or progesterone at the time.

The social effects of headaches

By charting the timing of headaches with hormonal fluctuations and menstrual bleeding, they may become predictable. Sufferers plan their professional and social lives around the headache times. It is particularly difficult for women with young children, who lack a family support network, as they often find it impossible to rest. The 21st century career woman, who needs to be performing at top level may find it difficult to compete when functional disorders associated with 'hormones' or 'menstruation' are still often wrongly minimised at 'psychosomatic'. This typical super-achiever and perfectionist will try to battle on, not admitting to her peers that she is unwell with a cyclical vulnerability that could make her less productive than a man.

Treatment of Hormonal Headaches

Women who find that hormonal headaches can be alleviated and prevented feel a relief akin to being 'sprung' from prison. If you refresh your memory with Diagram 7, it becomes clear that if we can prevent the blood levels of the sex hormones from falling, we can stop the trigger factor for a hormonal headache. Hormones can be given in several ways and, most importantly, need to be given every day to prevent blood hormone levels from falling.

The Oral Contraceptive Pill

Many migraine/vascular headache sufferers are unable to tolerate the oral contraceptive pill (OCP), as it can aggravate the frequency and severity of migraines or occasionally bring them on for the first time, while others find that the OCP does indeed effectively reduce hormonal-vascular type headaches. So the OCP can be unpredictable in its effect on headaches and it can be necessary to simply try it and see how you go. However severe migraine sufferers should totally avoid the OCP as it may increase the risk of strokes. The mini pill or 'progesterone only pill' is an exception and is usually well tolerated by migraineurs.

If the headache occurs only during menstruation in a woman on the OCP, it is necessary to give a low dose of oestrogen during the seven-day pill break (or seven days of sugar pills) between pill cycles. These could be tablets of oestradiol 2mg daily or an oestrogen patch or cream given during the seven-day break and your local doctor could prescribe this.

The OCP should be stopped immediately if it causes migraines associated with visual disturbances, such as blurred vision, flashing lights or golden lights or neurological problems, such as clumsiness, weakness, numbness or pins and needles in the limbs. In such cases, the risk of stroke (brain haemorrhage) is increased, especially in women over the age of 35.

MARIA'S CHART

CODE:
M = Menstrual bleeding
H = Headache
Maria has a 5-day bleeding cycle every 32 days
Ovulation occurs 14 days before menstrual bleeding starts.

	September	October	November	December
1	H			
2				
3		H		
4			H	
5				H
6				
7				
8				
9				
10				
11				
12				
13				
14	H			
15	M H	H		
16	M	H		
17	M H	M H	H	
18	M	M	M H	
19	M	M	M	H
20	H	M H	M H	M H
21		M	M H	M
22		H	M H	M H
23		H	H	M
24				M
25				
26				
27				
28				
29				
30				
31				

Natural Oestrogen

In women not requiring oral contraception, the natural forms of oestrogen can be given with the aim of maintaining constant oestrogen blood levels. If you have had a hysterectomy, this is a simple matter and natural oestrogen can be given in the form of the oestrogen patch or cream.

Life is a bit more complicated for those among us, who still have a uterus, in which case it is necessary to balance oestrogen with some type of progestogen. One possibility is to take the natural oestrogen every day without a break and along with this, take a progestogen such as Provera or Duphaston 5mg to 10mg daily for fourteen days every month. The progestogen given in this cyclical fashion will bring on a regular menstrual bleed. If you wish to avoid any menstrual bleeding the progestogen is taken every day.

If the headaches still occur at the time of menstruation, it is then possible to avoid menstruation altogether by taking both progestogen and natural oestrogen every day. This practice has been found to be effective and safe. If the synthetic progestogen aggravates your mood disorder you can replace it with capsules containing natural progesterone in a dose of at least 200mg daily.

I often emphasise, "Every woman is an individual" and what works for one woman, may not work for another. This is definitely true when it comes to hormone therapy and there will be a significant percentage of women, who find that oestrogen in all forms causes their headaches to worsen. In such cases, it may be worthwhile to withdraw all hormone therapy for three to six months and observe what happens to the headaches during a woman's own natural menstrual cycle. If the headaches still persist on a cyclical basis, it is then time to try natural progesterone by itself.

The observation that some women cannot tolerate oral forms of oestrogen and progesterone is common enough and is an interesting phenomenon. Many in this group of women will feel well taking oestrogen and/or progesterone if it is given in the form of creams. Hormones given this way are absorbed directly into the blood circulation and bypass the liver, thus having less effect on the function of the liver.

Many migraineurs find that they feel 'liverish' during their headache attacks with nausea and vomiting, or they complain that fatty or rich foods strain their liver and gall bladder and bring on a headache. These migraineurs need to reduce stress upon their livers in order to get their headaches under control.

For similar liverish reasons, migraineurs are wise to avoid all but the smallest amounts of alcohol and consume a liver-friendly diet. This diet is abundant in fresh vegetables and fruits (especially salads), whole grains, legumes, seeds, nuts and fish. Raw juicing will produce enormous benefits often leading to a huge reduction in the frequency and severity of headaches. A good juice for the liver consists of red apple, cabbage, carrot and a small amount of red onion and ginger root. For more great healing juice recipes see my book titled "Raw Juices can save your Life." The regular use of a magnesium supplement (4 tablets daily) and a good liver tonic can prevent many headaches.

Fatty or deep-fried foods and foods containing tyramine (red wine, beer, chocolate, Lima and Italian beans, mature cheeses, chicken liver & raisins) and monosodium glutamate are best avoided.

All migraineurs should endeavour to increase their daily water intake to around two to three litres, preferably bottled spring water or purified water. This simple measure alone can greatly reduce the frequency of headaches.

Treatment of an Acute Migraine

The key to success with an acute migraine lies in striking the attack on the head, so to speak, with measures being taken at the first hint of the migraine's onslaught.

Drug Approach

Preparations containing the drug ergotamine can be excellent in stopping the development of a migraine, as they prevent the blood vessels from swelling and throbbing. Ergotamine must be taken at the first sign of the migraine and is versatile being available as tablets, injections or suppositories. If ergotamine causes nausea, simply reduce the dosage or take it in suppository form. Some women find that one-half to one-third of a suppository of an ergotamine preparation, such as Cafergot, is enough to do the trick.

Ergotamine should be taken together with a painkiller, such as Aspalgin (aspirin + codeine) or Mersyndol. A tablet or suppository to stop nausea and vomiting may be essential, eg Stemetil or Maxolon. Many women find the group of drugs known as serotonin agonists ((examples of which are sumatriptan (Imigran) and naratriptan (Naramig)) highly effective in stopping an acute migraine. These drugs are available in the form of tablets or nasal spray.

Other Strategies

Non-drug approaches for the early stages of an acute migraine or cluster headache may be effective. I have had success giving intravenous vitamin C in one litre of mineral solution and, in cases of dehydration, 2 litres intravenously may be required. Clinical studies have shown that the inhalation of medical oxygen via a face mask can be up to 80% effective in relieving a migraine or cluster headache.

You can ask your local doctor about the availability of medical oxygen. He may have a cylinder in his surgery or may be able to fill in the necessary paperwork so that you can hire a cylinder of oxygen for use in your own home.

Headaches and Pregnancy

The vast majority of migraineurs are free of headaches after the first six weeks of pregnancy because of the very high levels of oestrogen and progesterone circulating in their blood stream. During pregnancy, the very high levels of progesterone cause relaxation of all the ligaments in the pelvis, joints and spine. Occasionally, the ligaments in the neck relax excessively causing the head to be unduly mobile upon the neck. This may result in unaccustomed headaches and even migraines, especially in the mornings, as the head may have twisted in relation to the neck during sleep.

This happened to a friend of mine, who suffered terrible headaches for the first time in her life during her first pregnancy. She consulted many doctors to no avail and finally came across a chiropractor, who told her to wear a firm foam rubber collar (cervical collar) to support her neck during sleep. From that point on, she never had a morning headache, which was indeed fortunate as she has had three more children. Cervical collars can be purchased from your local pharmacy.

CHAPTER 7

Postnatal Depression

Depression after childbirth, known as postnatal depression, is a common problem in modern society affecting up to 40% of young mothers. It may also be referred to as post-partum or puerperal depression and the most important thing for women to realise is that, if it is correctly diagnosed, it can be treated effectively with quick results. Postnatal depression may rear its ugly head any time during the first year after the baby's birth and inflict itself upon the most unsuspecting and unlikely candidates. It is just as likely to occur in women who have spent years in infertility clinics trying desperately to have a baby, as it is in those women, whose well ordered lives have been interrupted with an unwanted pregnancy.

There are three types of postnatal mood disorders, which are distinct in their features and require different treatment. It is helpful to look at the features of these three different types.

The Maternity Blues

This is sometimes called the 'post-partum blues' or the 'third day blues' and is just about as common as 'lovers blues', so much so that some clever guitarist should write a 12-bar blues song to play over the radio to offer solace to those tearful new mothers. Postnatal wards in maternity hospitals are sometimes called the 'weeping wards,' as at any one time, about 50% to 80% of its inpatients will be feeling overly emotional and excessively tearful.

Thankfully, maternity blues don't last too long and are generally not severe, followed by a spontaneous return to a normal, happy emotional state about 14 days after childbirth. This transient change in the emotional personality does not require medication and will pass with support, rest and reassurance.

If the birth has been prolonged or difficult, the new mother is often physically and mentally drained, feeling very anxious that she will not cope with the baby's needs and this can precipitate anxious and tearful moments, as can breastfeeding problems if they are not handled tactfully and patiently.

The nursery and medical staff should take great pains to try to accommodate the wishes of the new mother regarding the way she wants to spend the first few postnatal days with her baby, as things that may appear tiny and inconsequential to others, may seem vitally important to her. Doctors and nurses must realise that a new mother is vulnerable, dependent and often highly emotional, in need of support and sensitivity from those looking after her.

I remember an older mother coming to see me nine months after the birth of her second child, complaining of depression, anxiety and insomnia. She told me that she was haunted by the memory of the suturing of her episiotomy (vaginal cut) immediately after the birth of her baby. Her own obstetrician had been unavailable and his locum doctor had been called in at 3 am to do the stitching. This doctor had complained bitterly about his disturbed sleep and had joked with the nursing staff about his drunken weekend. He had refused to allow the mother to cuddle and breastfeed the baby immediately before he began stitching the vaginal tear, which had taken a full forty minutes. This woman found the doctor and staff totally insensitive and had longed for a quiet romantic twenty minutes with her baby immediately after birth. This patient was very angry and resentful, and being unable to express this to the doctor, she had turned it inside upon herself resulting in depression.

The sudden hormonal withdrawal during the first 24 hours after birth (see Diagram 8 page 75) is partly responsible for the third-day blues. This drop in hormones may also cause a migraine, an increase in general aches and pains and, occasionally in susceptible women, a flair up of arthritis, auto immune disorders or an asthma attack. These physical discomforts require specific treatment as they only add to the feelings of vulnerability and dependency in these early postnatal days.

Puerperal Psychosis

The second type of postnatal mood disorder is called puerperal psychosis and is a severe mental imbalance that needs urgent medical treatment. This type is vastly different to the common and mild maternity blues and, thankfully, is relatively rare occurring in only 2 to 3 cases per 1000 births.

Puerperal psychosis usually has a sudden and dramatic onset, manifesting within the first two to three weeks after childbirth and may occur as early as several hours after birth. It produces a total change in the mental state with thoughts and emotions becoming jumbled, frenzied, confused and irrational. The helpless victim of this psychosis becomes totally out of touch with reality, being tormented and preoccupied with weird thoughts that may cause her to behave in an agitated and paranoid manner. She may be subject to hallucinations of sight and smell, seeing and hearing voices and things that are not present, and imagining that she or her baby are in imminent and grave danger. Understandably, she may become disorientated and unable to sleep, eat or even care for her child.

Christine, a 31-year old single mother had had a normal pregnancy and easy vaginal delivery of a healthy baby and all seemed well as I wished her goodnight after checking her baby. The next morning when I arrived at her bedside, she had become a different person with an agitated and worried look upon her face. She insisted that the nurses had put a spell on her baby that made him susceptible to evil spirits and that her breast milk was poisonous. She wanted to purify the baby by putting him on a fast and giving him a bath in holy water. She asked me to urgently find a priest to exorcise the evil spirit out of her son with a cross and holy bible. Christine was continuously distracted by loud voices, although in reality her ward was quiet and almost empty. The nurses were unable to restrain or control this large, powerful woman and an urgent injection of tranquillising medication was required. It was nine months before Christine was able to care for her baby without constant supervision.

The most dangerous aspect of post-partum psychosis is that a sufferer may have compulsions or obsessions to harm herself or her baby and suicide and infanticide are not rare in this disorder.

One psychotic woman became so obsessed with the long shape of her baby's head that she was found trying to hammer it back into a rounder shape. Every year a case of severe puerperal psychosis tragically makes the newspaper headlines and we read that:

'Mother jumped out of hospital window with her baby'
'Mother stabs three children'
'Child suffocated by distraught mother'
'Two children and mother asphyxiated with car exhaust'

These tragedies should not occur and, if society, families and professionals were more aware of the early stages of post-partum psychosis, life-saving emergency treatment could be given. It is incredible to think that governments spend billions of dollars trying to cure AIDS, cancer and heart disease, and yet post-partum psychosis, which is easier to prevent and cure than these diseases, receives very little funding or attention and these tragedies continue.

Obviously, these women need 24-hour observation in a security hospital environment and major tranquillising drugs. The mother cannot be left alone with the baby under any circumstances even in the safety of a mother and baby unit within the hospital or mothercraft centre.

Post-partum psychosis requires powerful tranquillising drugs. When the mother is discharged from hospital care, her behaviour and emotional state is still influenced by these drugs so that she is usually slow and unable to care for her baby by herself. Generally, she would take anything from several months to several years for complete recovery, although hormonal therapy with natural progesterone and nutritional supplements may shorten her illness.

She, or her family, should be instructed to keep a menstrual calendar to check for pre-menstrual deteriorations in her mental state and once she is stable, an attempt can be made to reduce her tranquillisers. She may require extra natural progesterone to control pre-menstrual exacerbations of her psychosis.

Postnatal Depression

This illness falls in between the maternity blues and post-partum psychosis, being more severe that the former and less incapacitating and destructive than the latter. Postnatal depression is really a mixed bag of problems that varies in the type of symptoms, their severity and duration. Postnatal depression is very common and up to 40% of women are affected to some degree. The symptoms of postnatal depression may start any time during the twelve months after childbirth. Some people do not realise this, so postnatal depression may not be recognised for what it is, especially if it begins as long as six months after childbirth. Most commonly, it lasts for several months, but up to one in five women with postnatal depression are still feeling unwell twelve months after child birth.

What are the symptoms of postnatal depression?

The symptoms may include the following:

1. Psychological Symptoms

Depression, sadness, irritability, anxiety, loss of confidence, excessive worrying, panic attacks, feelings of unworthiness, anger, resentment, guilt, irrational fears, obsessions, excessive sleepiness or inability to sleep, emotional desolation with lack of feeling for the baby, rejection of the baby or excessive attachment to the baby, feeling spaced out, confusion, reduced intellectual and mental function, preoccupation with death, suicidal thoughts and/or desires to harm the baby.

2. Physical Symptoms

Light-headed feelings, low blood sugar levels, muscle aches and pains with flu-like feelings, headaches, increased or decreased appetite, eating binges with sugar and junk foods, increased or decreased weight, constipation and extreme exhaustion. There may be an aggravation of pre-existing diseases such as auto-immune disease.

Some mothers are too ashamed and feel too guilty to complain that they are depressed, and they subconsciously convert their emotional stress into physical symptoms. For instance, a young mother with masked depression may pay frequent visits to her doctor for minor physical complaints, such as fatigue or a crying colicky or vomiting baby. If the doctor cannot find any physical signs of abnormality, he should look deeper, as the mother may be desperate for emotional help but cannot ask, as she does not want to be stigmatised as an inadequate mother.

It is vital that women with postnatal depression receive early and adequate treatment because if it is allowed to progress, it may have a devastating effect and produce marital conflict and deterioration in the relationship between the depressed mother and her baby. The babies of depressed mothers are more likely to suffer with feeding and sleeping difficulties and develop mental problems. Professor of Psychiatry at Monash University, Professor Bruce Tong, has found that such babies may become either emotionally distant or detached from their mothers, or more clinging and demanding and unable to be soothed. Professor Tong found that if the depression continued for twelve months, the baby may become irritable with reduced concentration or show less interest in surrounding activities than the babies of non-depressed mothers. If the depression should become deeper, a mother could get to the stage of not coping and may be at risk of harming the baby. She may shake or spank the baby excessively, or feel like throwing it on the floor. The guilty feelings engendered by this behaviour make it even more difficult for her to ask for help. A vicious circle develops and it is easy for social isolation to occur.

3. Sexuality and Postnatal Depression

Women with postnatal depression often have a loss of interest in sex and may even become sexually frigid to the point of being annoyed or repulsed by the advances of their partner. This may be due to a combination of their loss of sex hormones, physical exhaustion, side effects from anti-depressant medication or inadequate contraception, especially if the birth has been painful or traumatic.

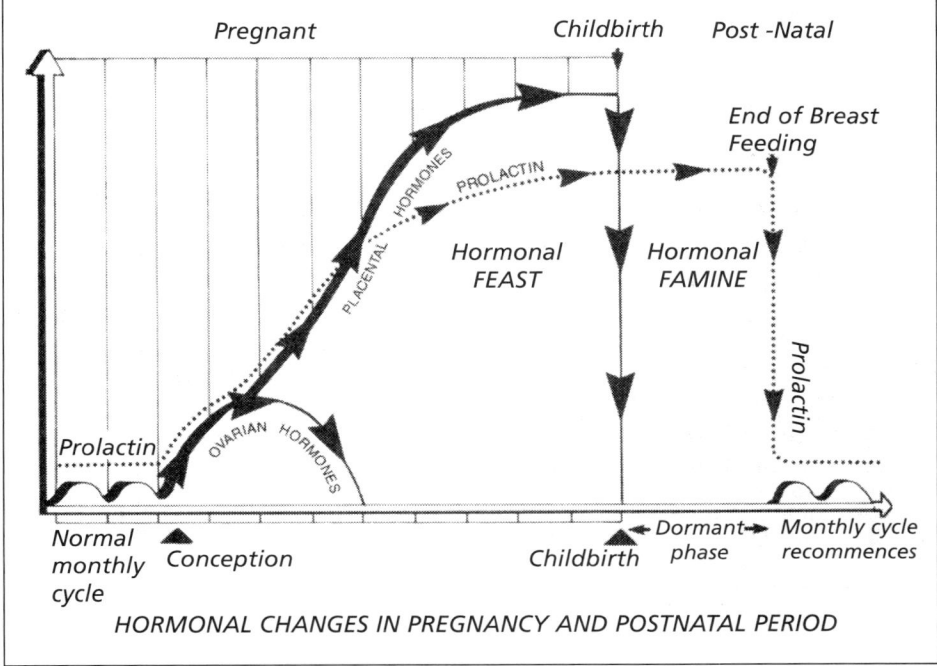

DIAGRAM 8

HORMONAL CHANGES IN PREGNANCY AND POSTNATAL PERIOD

Lindy had given birth to a bouncing baby boy in February and all was going well until postnatal depression insidiously set in during the following May. She stopped breastfeeding and her first menstruation, which was heralded by severe pre-menstrual syndrome, arrived in June. She felt some relief after her menstruation began, although the following months were stressful, as she was exhausted and totally disinterested in sex, which made her husband irritable and cranky. In September, she approached her doctor, as she was worried about depression, sexual frigidity, absent periods and continuing milk from her breasts, even though she had stopped breastfeeding in May.

The presence of inappropriate breast milk production in the absence of breastfeeding is called galactorrhoea and is often associated with an excessive production of the lactation hormone called 'Prolactin' from the pituitary gland.

Lindy's doctor told her that her 'menstrual clock' situated in the hypothalamus (see page 16) was not working properly and when he measured the blood level of the hormone prolactin, it was way too high. Once he had ruled out the possibility of a pituitary tumour, he started Lindy on a course of Bromocriptine (Parlodel) tablets to reduce her prolactin levels to normal.

If the prolactin levels are too high, the ovaries remain in a dormant state and do not produce the female sex hormones oestrogen and progesterone, and so regular menstruation does not occur. This is why full-time regular breastfeeding acts as a good contraceptive especially in poor countries.

Lindy took the Bromocriptine tablets for eight weeks, and once her prolactin levels came down to normal, her breast milk dried up, her menstruation returned and she began once more to feel sexually alive.

Prolactin is not the only hormone that may be out of balance postnatally and if you are suffering with loss of libido or sexual difficulties during your first postnatal year, it is wise to have a blood test. This test should check your levels of the sex steroid hormones, oestrogen and testosterone, as these are largely responsible for creating sexual desire. Also, ask your doctor to check the levels of free testosterone and the Free Androgen Index (FAI), as it is the free or unbound component of testosterone that is active in your body. The best measure of free male hormones is the 'Free Androgen Index' or FAI, which is easily measured in a simple blood test and is often found to be very low in women with poor libido or sexual frigidity. (see page 177)

Some women find that the combined oral contraceptive pill is not suiting them postnatally, as it may greatly reduce sexual desire, as well as cause depression to persist. In such cases, you may try a progesterone-only contraceptive pill, also known as a 'mini pill' and if this does not improve matters, consider using condoms, an intra-uterine contraceptive device or a vaginal diaphragm.

4. Physical Exhaustion

During the first six months after childbirth, women may suffer with fatigue and lethargy, craving sleep and unable to get through the routine chores. If blood loss at birth was excessive, iron deficiency is common and, especially if breastfeeding, the body's iron stores quickly become depleted if supplemental iron is not given. Iron supplements can be taken on an empty stomach with citrus fruit or vitamin C to aid absorption.

Other mineral deficiencies are not uncommon at this time and supplements of calcium, zinc, magnesium and selenium can be a wonderful aid to boost flagging energy reserves.

Your body is going through enormous physiological changes during the first six postnatal weeks - the blood volume diminishes and the uterus shrinks back to its non-pregnant size. If you are breastfeeding, particularly in a hot climate, dehydration may cause profound exhaustion and you should drink at least three litres of fluid daily in the form of purified water and/or herbal teas.

Raw vegetable juices are vitally important to restore your energy levels and I recommend that you aim to make yourself a raw juice combination of fruits and vegetables (in season varieties are best) every day. Raw juicing is a great way to increase the quantity and quality of your breast milk.

If you find that your skin and hair become very dry and your metabolism slows down, ask your doctor to check the function of your thyroid gland, as it may have become temporarily underactive. The function of the thyroid gland can be improved with supplemental selenium, cold pressed flaxseed oil, spirulina, a good mineral supplement (such as Calcium Complete) and culinary seaweeds (sea vegetables) such as arame, wakame, kombu, nori and kelp.

Some women, who have been subjected to excessive and continuous stress postnatally, may find that the cause of their fatigue is a temporary under activity of their adrenal glands known as **'adrenal exhaustion'**. This will gradually recover with increased rest, raw juicing and a good multi-vitamin and mineral formulation.

Severe dysfunction of the pituitary and adrenal glands can occur subsequent to very heavy blood loss at the time of childbirth. This will manifest as extreme fatigue, dizziness and a failure to recommence regular menstruation at the appropriate time. If you have these symptoms, I highly recommend that you see a specialist endocrinologist who will check the function of your pituitary and adrenal glands.

Margaret's story

Margaret had lost nearly a litre of blood from a tear in her cervix during the rapid vaginal birth of her daughter. Despite a blood transfusion, she still felt exhausted four months after birth and complained that she had lost all her old energy. She felt dizzy and light-headed and continually craved sugar and carbohydrates.

I found that Margaret's blood pressure and blood sugar levels were very low and that her blood cortisone levels were at the lower limit of normal in both the mornings and evenings.

The adrenal glands produce the hormone cortisone and other hormones involved in the control of blood sugar levels and blood pressure.

Margaret was not anaemic, as she was on iron supplements. I diagnosed 'adrenal gland exhaustion', which I reassured her would recover with rest and time. To speed up the adrenal recovery, I prescribed a daily regime of vitamin C with bioflavonoids 4000mg, vitamin E 500 I.U., Calcium Complete 2 tablets, Power Woman multi one tablet and Stoney Creek cold pressed flaxseed oil 2 tsp. I also encouraged her to do raw juicing everyday.

Margaret was encouraged to eat small frequent meals containing protein and raw fruits and vegetables. First-class protein and complex carbohydrates can be obtained by combining three of the following – grains, nuts, seeds and legumes at one meal. Other good sources of first-class protein are lean fresh meats, seafood, organic or free range chicken and eggs, and feta cheese.

After six weeks on her new diet and supplements, Margaret regained her old vitality. Her blood sugar and cortisone levels increased into the middle of the normal range and she was delighted that she no longer binged on chocolate and sweet biscuits.

Hormonal Changes in Pregnancy

In the non-pregnant woman, the regular monthly menstrual cycle is controlled by the hormonal rhythm regulator or 'hormonal clock' situated in the area of the brain called the hypothalamus. (Diagram 4 on page 16). Once conception occurs, around day 14 of the menstrual cycle, the production of oestrogen and progesterone from the ovaries increases to higher levels than those found in a non-pregnant woman. (see Diagram 8 on page 75). This early surge of ovarian hormones immediately after conception may induce nausea, fatigue and sore breasts even before the next period is missed. Some women may feel quite different and be sure that they are pregnant within several days after conception.

In early pregnancy, hormonal control is taken over by the placenta and foetus and the 'hormonal clock' in the hypothalamus becomes inactive until menstruation returns after childbirth. The cells surrounding the tiny embryo pump out the unique pregnancy hormone called 'human chorionic gonadotrophin' (HCG), which stimulates the ovaries to greatly increase their production of oestrogen and progesterone. During the first eight weeks of pregnancy, oestrogen and progesterone are mainly produced by the ovary but after this time, the placenta becomes dominant and behaves like a huge endocrine gland gradually increasing its manufacture of oestrogen and progesterone to enormous levels (see Diagrams 8&9). The placenta is very efficient and produces progesterone levels up to 300 times higher and oestrogen levels up to 50 times higher than the maximum levels found during a non-pregnant menstrual cycle. During pregnancy the pituitary gland produces large quantities of prolactin hormone and the adrenal glands double their output of cortisol. Thus, during pregnancy, we could say that women enjoy a 'hormonal feast' and this is why most women feel so well mentally and physically during pregnancy. One of my patients, who has pre-menstrual syndrome commented that during pregnancy, she feels like Superwoman and rediscovers the woman she is meant to be. She made me laugh when she told me that she was considering applying for a full-time job as a surrogate mother.

The Hormonal Drama of Childbirth

Within hours after the delivery of the baby and placenta, there is a large and precipitous fall in the levels of the sex hormones so that only tiny amounts of these hormones are found in the mother's body. What has taken nine months to develop is suddenly withdrawn, and a woman passes from a 'hormonal feast' to a 'hormonal famine' in a matter of several hours. Progesterone disappears completely by the seventh day after birth, and oestrogen levels become very low in the same time span. Synonymous with this, the pituitary gland pumps out large amounts of prolactin to produce lactation, and the ovaries enter into a dormant or resting phase. (see Diagram 8 page 75) The high levels of prolactin ensure that the ovaries remain unresponsive and dormant and thus the levels of the ovarian sex hormones oestrogen and progesterone remain very low until a woman decides to stop breastfeeding. Then prolactin levels reduce to normal levels. Thus, the length of the dormant phase of the ovaries varies from several weeks to several years depending upon the duration of breastfeeding and high Prolactin levels. During the dormant postnatal phase of the ovaries, the menstrual clock in the hypothalamus is switched off and remains so until menstruation returns.

The hypothalamus also influences mood, sleep, appetite and day/night body rhythms. Because these basic body functions are often disturbed in women with postnatal depression, many experts believe that the hypothalamic control centres may be at fault.

When one understands the precipitous hormonal drama of childbirth, it is easy to understand that these hormonal changes can initiate maternity blues, post-partum psychosis or postnatal depression. Indeed, it is truly amazing that most women come through these hormonal upheavals without complaining and they should be commended and praised for this.

The Treatment of Postnatal Depression

It is true to say that sometimes the treatment of postnatal depression appears somewhat confused with different doctors having very different approaches to helping a woman with depression after childbirth. This is because the treatment of postnatal depression falls in between the three different medical specialities of obstetrics, psychiatry and endocrinology. This is of little comfort to the depressed and ailing woman, who only wishes to find the quickest and safest way out of her desolation.

It is reassuring to know that postnatal depression can be completely cured, provided it is recognised and treated early after birth. Furthermore, postnatal depression can be prevented from recurring after subsequent pregnancies, provided once again treatment is given immediately after birth. There are many women who do not realise this and are too frightened to have further children. Dr Katharina Dalton has found that without preventative treatment, the chance of postnatal depression recurring after subsequent births is 2 out of 3 (Ref 3).

Hormonal Treatment

Progesterone

Treatment of postnatal depression with natural progesterone is rather controversial among the experts. However, large studies of women with postnatal depression in the UK conducted by Dr Dalton (Ref 3) have found injections and suppositories/pessaries of progesterone to be fairly successful.

Dr Dalton found that the natural recurrence rate of 2 in 3 women for postnatal depression could be reduced to less than 1 in 10 if progesterone was given immediately after childbirth. Dr Dalton believes that after birth, the precipitous fall in progesterone to negligible levels, initiates the depression, and thus, if progesterone injections are given to reduce this fall, the depression will be lessened or avoided. She recommends that natural progesterone is given as an intra-muscular injection in a dose of 100mg daily for the first seven days after birth. In Australia, natural progesterone injections are only available in the form of Proluton 25mg ampoules. Thus, you would need four of these 25mg ampoules to be drawn up into one syringe, which could be injected deeply into the buttocks once a day for seven days. The first of these progesterone injections must be given at the completion of birth before the symptoms of postnatal depression begin, and Dr Dalton says that the anti-depressant effect of this progesterone is greatly lessened if the injections are delayed until symptoms of depression are present.

Natural progesterone is very safe, does not interfere with breastfeeding and does not affect the newborn babe adversely. The main drawbacks of progesterone injections are their expense and the fact that oily injections are uncomfortable and indeed can be painful if given incorrectly.

According to Dr Dalton after the first seven postnatal days, the progesterone injections are replaced with progesterone vaginal pessaries or rectal suppositories, which are given in a dose of 2 x 200mg pessaries twice daily, providing a total daily progesterone dose of 800mg. These pessaries/suppositories are continued until the moods have stabilised. They can then be replaced by progesterone cream, troches or capsules and these can be continued until the natural menstrual periods return. This means that breastfeeding mothers may need to continue them for many months.

These days the regime of injections that Dr Dalton originally recommended can usually be replaced with natural progesterone creams or troches from the outset, which most women find much more convenient and less expensive than progesterone injections.

DIAGRAM 9

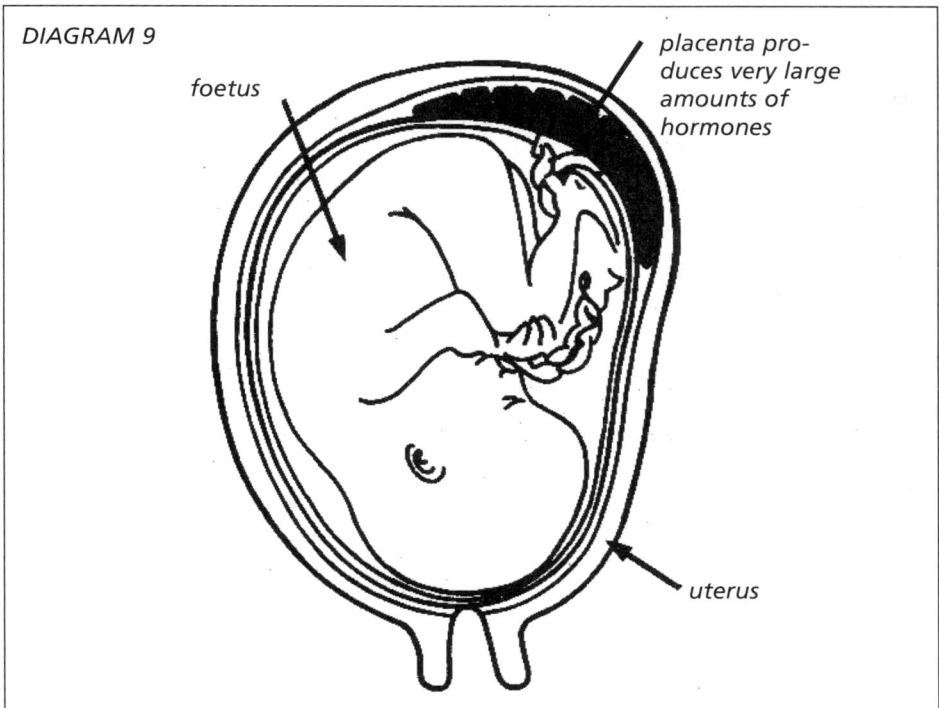

foetus

placenta pro-
duces very large
amounts of
hormones

uterus

Other hormones used in postnatal depression

For postnatal depression in older women, or if it is associated with a loss of libido and marital discord, the temporary use of natural oestrogen and testosterone can be very effective in elevating the mood and energy levels and in restoring sexual desire and pleasure. Oestrogen should not be given during the first six weeks after childbirth, as there is an increased risk of thrombosis (blood clots) at this time. Furthermore, oestrogen and/or testosterone cannot be used in breastfeeding women, as they reduce the milk supply and these hormones can adversely affect the baby. Natural oestrogen and/or testosterone can be started six weeks after childbirth in women, who do not want to breastfeed and who are active and mobile. Adequate contraception in the form of the progesterone-only mini pill, a low dose contraceptive pill, condoms, a vaginal diaphragm or an intra-uterine device (IUD) is necessary. If you decide to try natural oestrogen and/or testosterone to overcome your postnatal depression, I suggest you receive it in the form of creams, which contain a combination of natural oestrogen, progesterone and testosterone. Blood tests to check your hormonal levels can be helpful in deciding the dose and choice of hormones that is best for you.

Drug Treatments for postnatal depression

Bromocriptine (Parlodel)

This drug lowers the level of the pituitary hormone prolactin and so smartly brings breastfeeding to an end. It may be tried in women with postnatal depression and poor libido, who do not want to breastfeed. Parlodel will speed up the return of ovulation and menstruation and thus normal levels of oestrogen and progesterone will return in the monthly cyclical pattern. This should relieve depression and poor libido due to the very low levels of sex hormones found in the normal postnatal months. (Diagram 8 on page 75)

Anti-Depressant Drugs

Some women with postnatal depression definitely need anti-depressant medication and we do not have a test that will tell us if your depression will respond to hormones, or anti-depressants, or if it will require both. Thus, patience is required from both the doctor and the patient and although a little trial and error may occur, effective relief is sure to be found. There are different types of anti-depressant drugs and your doctor should know which type suits your depression the best.

The Tricyclic anti-depressant drugs have been used for many years to treat all types of depression and are particularly effective if the depression is associated with anxiety, worried thoughts, panic attacks, excessive mental activity, reduced appetite and poor sleep. It is best to start with small doses, as many women will respond to these, and it is possible to continue breastfeeding if you are only taking small to moderate doses of the Tricyclic anti-depressant drugs. If your doctor finds it necessary to increase the dose of these drugs, do not be alarmed, as this is only temporary, and these drugs are very safe. Examples of the Tricyclic antidepressant drugs are Tofranil, Sinequan, Doxepin and Prothiaden.

The Monoamine Oxidase Inhibitors (MAOIs) are drugs which prevent your enzymes from breaking down the brain's neuro-transmitters and, in particular, those called the biogenic amines, which are powerful anti-depressants. Examples of the MAOI drugs are Parnate and Aurorix. The Monoamine Oxidase Inhibitor drugs are powerful anti-depressants and may be very helpful for you if your postnatal depression is associated with a complete loss of energy, mental dullness, apathy and loss of interest in your family and surroundings. The advantages of the MAOI drugs are that they work quickly and do not cause drowsiness as a side effect and indeed, they wake you up, so that they should be taken on awakening and no later than 3 pm, and definitely not at night.

The group of drugs known as Serotonin Re-uptake Inhibitors (SRIs) are excellent anti-depressants and balance out the moods and normalise sleep patterns. Examples of the SRI drugs are Cipramil, Prozac, Zoloft and Aropax. Possible side effects of the SRI drugs are a reduction in sex drive and a small gain in weight.

Anti-depressant drugs are often needed for twelve months or more to really cure postnatal depression. Once the depression has lifted completely, the drugs are slowly withdrawn over a period of several months, which does not present a problem, as antidepressant drugs are not addictive or habit forming. In many women best results are obtained by using a combination therapy of natural progesterone and anti-depressant drugs.

Stopping Medications

This should always be done gradually with small reductions in the dose being made in two-weekly or monthly steps. This applies if you are taking anti-depressant drugs or progesterone. The reduction should be made at the end of menstrual bleeding and not during the pre-menstrual phase. Anti-depressant drugs and natural hormones are not habit forming, which means that once the illness has passed, a gradual reduction in their dosage is not problematic and should not result in rebound depression.

Be Prepared

It is not wise to first consider postnatal depression once it has hit you. You and your family should discuss this possibility during the pregnancy so that you are all able to recognise the first signs of this illness. If you have already suffered with a bout of postnatal depression, make sure that during your next pregnancy, you discuss all your treatment options with your family, general practitioner and obstetrician while you are still objective about it. If progesterone may be necessary, it can be pre-arranged by your general practitioner and obstetrician to be available for you at the hospital immediately after birth.

Psychology and Postnatal Depression

This is a huge subject and it is not possible in a book about hormones to physically fit it all in. The reader is recommended to read the book, The New Mother Syndrome by Carol Dix and published by Allen & Unwin to explore the psychological effects of having a baby.

I myself have never had children and so do not really feel qualified to tackle the psychological consequences that babies may provoke in our lives. I've left this to my sister, Madeleine, to tell you how she felt hormonally, mentally and emotionally after childbirth.

Surviving the First Year After Childbirth

By Madeleine McRae, mother of three happy beautiful talented children

Being a woman is a fantastic gift. We have the opportunity to experience life growing within us, giving birth and then sustaining that new life and watching it grow. We become intrinsically linked with the process of the cycle of life. Pretty amazing stuff! So who said it was gong to be easy! As women, we are by nature intuitive and instinctive beings and our hormonal cycle is influenced by the lunar phases, which have great power over many of the processes of nature.

Surviving the changes that befall us during pregnancy and lactation is no menial task and one we are definitely not educated for. It is imperative that we trust our own intuition and believe in our own ability, as every child is different, and if we can really 'tune in' to that child and follow our instincts, it will all unfold as it is meant to do.

The most important thing is your attitude. Don't cling to preconceived ideas and concepts about how it is going to be, or how it should be. You may feel great and have an angelic baby or you may feel terrible and have a screaming baby that never sleeps. Accept it and flow with it, or life is going to be frustrating, bewildering and beset with negativity and unfulfilment. All the above is easy to say and difficult to achieve. I learnt from my first child to let go within the first week of our life together. What does 'let go' mean? For me it meant accepting that he was the kind of baby that never slept and breastfed every 1½ hours and screamed with colic and took more than I had to give. What happened to my life? It became non-existent!

Thankfully my next two children were much easier to cope with, especially after having a first child like this. So, having accepted that he was an abominable baby, (who has since grown into an amazing adult), I had to work out how I was going to survive the first year.

I was very very tired. Absolutely exhausted would be more truthful, and I felt frightened, vulnerable and full of self-doubt. None of my family had any idea how to cope with him, my husband included! My husband's first thought at the time of birth was "That's very nice, but can we put him back now!"

Thinking of survival I went out and bought a king-size bed and put him in between myself and my husband, because when he woke at night, I found it easy to put him on the breast and feed him lying down. We got a lot more sleep that way. In a word, I learnt very quickly how to totally surrender. He bathed with me or my husband and I bought a snugly to carry him around in, and finally life began to settle down a little. He became like an "extra limb", always hanging there somewhere. Everyone tried to tell me I was doing the wrong thing, spoiling him and making a rod for my own back. I just trusted what we had going, and then it became far more enjoyable.

Having no time left for you can be very challenging – a bit like a prison sentence! I mean washing your hair becomes a luxury and when one of your fantasies becomes sleeping six hours through without interruption – you know you've got it bad.

Life becomes an endless saga of changing nappies, washing, cleaning, breastfeeding and just keeping baby happy. Ah! It's called the joys of motherhood.

One may suffer from -

Looking in the mirror at the 5 kilograms you still need to lose – here's my tip -just keep breastfeeding and it will gradually go.
Isolation and lack of adult company. Your friends find it all a bit boring and it

becomes difficult to get out of the house.

Total loss of your sexual identity. How can you feel sexy when you don't ever get to do anything that stimulates that part of your psyche?

Loss of personal achievements other than motherhood.

Loss of freedom. Will you ever be able to have a phone conversation without harassment again? What happened to those long baths and lazy lunches with friends?

Tiredness and anxiety over baby's health problems (of which there are many), stitches, sore nipples, mastitis, haemorrhoids, weakness. The list is endless.

Feeling alone, misunderstood and discontented.

All women will experience some of the above emotions and let downs and if they don't, they must be numb or lying to themselves. It is natural to feel like this and it's not wrong; it's not a sign of failure! Our body's hormonal cycle is still in fluctuation and we had so many ideas and romantic notions that have no doubt taken a beating.

I remember looking out the window and just waiting for my mother to arrive every morning after my third child was born, which she did, thank God for six weeks. We need somebody understanding to help us through this initial phase and we need our husbands to realise that if there is nothing left of ourselves for us, how can there be any left for them. We need support and not extra demands. With time, we reclaim our identity on all levels and what an incredible joy it is. It's like being reborn.

Being a mother has taught me the value of time and I have had to learn so many lessons about myself that I might otherwise have run away from. It is the greatest love you'll ever know and the greatest sacrifice you'll ever make. Where would the world be without relationships like grandmother to granddaughter, daughter to mother, mother to son etc?

Remember, don't take yourself too seriously and don't expect too much of yourself. Take it day by day and trust in yourself totally because then all things become possible.

CHAPTER 8

Contraception – and how it can affect your hormones

The Oral Contraceptive Pill (OCP)

So far, this book has dealt with how your own hormones can affect you and yet four out of every five Western women in their mid-30s either take or have taken at some time, the Oral Contraceptive Pill (OCP). The OCP effectively suppresses the natural production of sex hormones from the ovary. The combined OCP contains synthetic oestrogen and synthetic progesterone (progestagen) and these hormones switch off the menstrual clock in the hypothalamus and pituitary gland. This means that the ovaries do not receive a message from the pituitary gland to produce a mature egg, so ovulation does not occur. Without ovulation the ovaries do not produce their normal quota of natural oestrogen and progesterone.

The synthetic hormones comprising the various brands of oral contraceptive pills (OCPs) are primarily designed to prevent ovulation and thus conception but they may also exert both favourable and unfavourable effects upon a woman. In this chapter, we shall explore these effects.

Today's modern low-dose OCP is a very efficient and safe form of contraception. The triphasic OCPs (eg. Triquilar or Triphasil) contain less hormones in one month's packet than was found in one tablet of the original OCP designed fifty years ago!

To help you put the risk of the OCP into perspective, taking a relatively high dose OCP (by today's standard) is no more dangerous than going for a one-hour drive in your car. In the context of the fact that the combined oral contraceptive pill is the most effective form of temporary contraception, its risks are offset by the risk to mother and child of unplanned and unwanted pregnancy or abortion.

The Different Types of Oral Contraceptive Pill

The Combined Oral Contraceptive Pill (OCP)

This contains both oestrogen and progesterone in synthetic forms and in varying amounts, depending on the brand. The synthetic oestrogen used in the pill is ethinyl oestradiol and the synthetic progesterones are norethisterone, levonorgestrel, gestodene or desogestrel. Unfortunately, natural hormones, as used in Hormone Replacement Therapy during the menopause, are not potent enough to prevent conception.

Of all the brands of combined OCPs available today, the triphasic OCPs, such as Triquilar, come closest to copying the natural menstrual cycle, as they deliver varying amounts of hormones at different times during the menstrual cycle. This means that over one complete cycle, the total amount of hormone ingested is less than that from an oral contraceptive pill, where the amount of hormone delivered is the same every day. The more modern progestogens found in some brands of the OCP are called desogestrel, gestodene and norgestimate. The advantage of these new generation progestogens, are that compared to the older progestogens (norethisterone and levonorgestrel), they have less tendency to produce an unfavourable effect upon the balance of the blood fats (cholesterol & triglycerides). Thus theoretically they should not increase the risk of cardiovascular disease as much as the older generation progestogens.

Yasmin is the brand name of a new OCP that contains a new type of progestogen called drospirenone combined with ethinyl estradiol. Drospirenone has a dual action; it will reduce excess sodium and water in the body while maintaining, and in some cases increasing, the level of the beneficial mineral potassium. The benefit of this action is that Yasmin may reduce the symptoms of premenstrual bloating, fluid retention and breast pain. However due to this effect, it is not suitable for women with kidney disease, liver disease or adrenal disease.

Yasmin also has no masculinising (androgenic) effect and indeed has shown some anti-androgenic action in clinical trials, which makes it a good choice for women who suffer from acne, excess facial hair and Polycystic Ovarian Syndrome.

The Progesterone Only Pill

The Progesterone Only Pill (POP) is also referred to as the 'mini pill'. It contains only one hormone in the form of synthetic progesterone and does not contain any oestrogen, which is the other sex hormone. Commonly prescribed brands of the POP are Micronor or Microlut. Because the POP contains such a small amount of hormone, it must be taken every day, at the same time each day and without any breaks. It needs to be taken at least three hours before sexual intercourse, so that if you have sex later at night, you would be safe to take it around 6pm each day. The POP provides such a low dose of hormone that it causes only very small changes in your metabolism and thus does not cause any of the potentially serious side effects (such as blood clots, strokes or high blood pressure) occasionally associated with the combined OCP. The POP does not increase your risk of cardiovascular disease or cancer.

Because of its safety, the POP is an ideal contraceptive for women over 45, who are worried that the combined OCP may increase their chances of cardiovascular disease. Women aged over 35 who smoke, and diabetics, migraine sufferers and those with high blood pressure, or women who get side effects from the combined OCP, are also good candidates for the POP. (see table on page 100). The POP is a suitable and safe contraceptive for breastfeeding women and women unable to take oestrogen for medical reasons, such as liver disease, severe varicose veins, blood clots or high blood pressure.

The POP has a pregnancy rate of around 4% and as such is not quite as reliable as the combined OCP, which has a failure rate of only around 1%. The POP is more suited to older women or breastfeeding mothers, whose fertility is less than that of younger or non-lactating women, who may fear the 4% failure rate is unacceptable.

The mini pill is safe and generally well tolerated although one in four women get annoying irregular menstruation and breakthrough bleeding. This may be too problematic for sportive, outdoor women, who like to control their menstrual cycle. Other women, who should avoid the POP are those with a history of ectopic pregnancy or pelvic inflammatory disease, as the POP may increase your chances of ectopic pregnancy. An ectopic pregnancy is one occurring outside the uterus, usually in the uterine tubes.

What are the benefits of using the combined Oral Contraceptive Pill?

Many women think that the only benefit of the combined OCP is reliable protection against unwanted pregnancy and yet, it may also confer other benefits and may be prescribed to help women with various gynaecological and hormonal problems. Let us take a look at some of the other effects of the OCP in your body.

1. Your menstrual bleeding will usually be controlled and regular. If you prefer to miss a period because of some special event, this is easy to plan, simply by skipping the usual seven day break (or substitute sugar pills) between pill packets. In the vast majority of women on the combined OCP, menstrual bleeding becomes lighter and less painful and a complete relief of period cramps may often result.

2. Your chances of pelvic infection from certain bacteria (such as gonor-

rhoea) may be less, although this does not apply to all venereal infections and, in particular, the pill does not reduce your chances of infection with the wart virus, herpes virus or chlamydia.

3. Your chances of forming cysts on your ovaries will be 50% to 80% less and mid-cycle pains due to ovulation will usually be cured by the combined OCP. Mild cases of endometriosis can often by controlled by the combined OCP with beneficial effects upon future fertility.

4. The combined pill may help some women with pre-menstrual syndrome or pre-menopausal symptoms due to imbalances or deficiencies in their own sex hormones. This is because it supplies a steady amount of synthetic hormones, which compensate for unpleasant hormonal highs and lows. Pre-menopausal women may find that their vaginal lubrication and sexual function is helped by the combined OCP and it helps to protect their bones against calcium loss. Once the menopause arrives, the OCP should be replaced with natural Hormone Replacement Therapy if a personal choice to continue with hormone therapy is made. If you are taking the OCP for contraception and think that you may be menopausal, it is necessary to stop the OCP for 3 months and then have a blood test to check to see if your hormones are at menopausal levels. If you have a blood test to check for menopause either while you are on the OCP, or immediately after stopping the OCP, the blood test results will be meaningless and inaccurate.

5. Many women will be delighted to know that specific brands of the OCP or a special 'tailor-made' combined OCP can cure acne, pimples, oily hair and reduce excessive facial and body hair.

The most effective brands of the OCP for achieving this are 'Diane' and 'Brenda.' These brands contain the hormones ethinyl oestradiol and cyproterone (Androcur) combined in one pill, and can dramatically improve hormonal types of acne. Diane is the most popular brand of OCP prescribed for this reason. Many women choose to take a brand of OCP that promotes feminine skin and hair if given the choice. If you suffer with more severe degrees of acne or superfluous hair, higher doses of Androcur can be taken concurrently with Diane or Brenda, at least initially. (Refer to chapter 10 for details). OCPs containing the progestogen called levonorgestrel can worsen acne, and more suitable progestogens are cyproterone, desogestrel, gestodene or drosperinone. The OCP may take up to 6 months to cure acne.

6. In women anxious about the small size of their breasts, the OCP, particularly brands with higher oestrogen content (around 50mcg of ethinyl oestradiol per tablet), often produces a desirable increase in breast size.

7. Many women with infrequent menstruation can benefit by taking the combined OCP. Women who often miss their periods for several months to six months at a time (a condition known as amenorrhoea) have a problem with the function of their ovaries or pituitary gland. They may have too little oestrogen production from their ovaries, especially if they are underweight or very sportive. Conversely they may have excessive oestrogen and male hormone production from their ovaries, especially if they are overweight with skin problems. Those with too little oestrogen run an increased risk of osteoporosis and fractures of the spine and hips, while those with too much oestrogen face an increased risk of uterine cancer. By correcting these hormonal imbalances, the combined OCP prevents osteoporosis and reduces the risk of uterine cancer, if taken regularly in women with infrequent menstruation. Of course, the combined oral contraceptive pill enables regular menstruation to occur. In women who do not need contraception, the use of natural progesterone can restore a regular menstrual cycle and bleeding pattern, and many women prefer to take natural progesterone over the OCP. If you have been taking the OCP for contraception and you suspect that you may be starting the menopause because you are getting close to the age of 50, you may not wish to continue taking the OCP because you prefer to use natural hormones. In such cases you will need to stop taking the OCP, wait for 3 months, and then have a blood test for menopause. If your FSH levels are over 25 on 2 separate occasions, you are menopausal and thus no longer need contraception. Blood tests for menopause are unreliable and inconclusive if they are done while you are still taking the OCP.

The Combined OCP and the risk of cancer

If you are on the combined OCP, you have less chance of developing cancer of the ovary and uterus and this protective effect lasts for approximately fifteen years after coming off the pill.

You will also have less chance of non-cancerous (benign) breast lumps. The effect of the OCP upon your risk of breast cancer is not so clear and may vary depending upon the age at which you started the pill and for how long you took it. (Ref 20)

The Harvard University study of over 120,000 nurses aged 30 to 55 published in the Journal of The National Cancer Institute, found no link between the use of the combined OCP and breast cancer, even in cases where the OCP was taken for an extended time. Studies of women aged less than 45, who had used the pill before the age of 25, have shown an increasing relative risk of breast cancer with years of pill use, especially in women, who have never given birth. (Ref 21). A Scandinavian study of 422 women aged less than 45, showed a trend of increased breast cancer risk with duration of OCP use, and an increased risk for eight or more years of use before the first pregnancy.

Two European studies have found an increased risk of breast cancer in women, who started the pill at an early age, but the United States Federal Drug Administration believes that existing evidence does not support a change in prescription and use of the combined OCP.

More research is needed to determine the risk of breast cancer associated with use of the combined OCP at a young age, because women, who have taken the pill when young, are only now reaching the age where the breast cancer risk is highest. This research should also examine the interaction of the pill with diet, exercise and lifestyle factors in determining its long-term effects upon cancer.

Young women should be told that there may be a slightly increased risk of breast cancer from long-term use of the combined OCP. This enables them to give valid informed consent when making choices in their method of contraception.

The effect of the combined OCP upon cancer of the cervix also needs more research, as one study has shown an increased incidence in women on the OCP, especially after ten years use, but cause and effect has not been proven. (Ref 22). A large multi-centre trial published by the World Health Organisation showed an increased risk of cervical cancer after 5 years of OCP use. It is not clear if this increased risk is directly due to the OCP, or if it is due to the concurrent increase in the prevalence of the venereal wart virus.

Thus, it is most important that all women on the OCP have regular annual pap smears.

Combined oral contraceptives probably increase the risk of primary liver cancer. This is not true for women who only use the OCP for a short time, but OCP use for eight years or more is associated with a fourfold increased risk. However, hepatitis B and C remain a far greater risk for liver cancer, than does the OCP.

Side Effects of the Combined OCP

When the OCP was first introduced over 40 years ago, its high doses of synthetic hormones were far more likely to induce side effects such as nausea, headaches, weight gain, high blood pressure, blood clots, and strokes than today's low dose OCPs are. Indeed, the original OCP was more suited to an elephant than a woman! We are still searching for the ideal contraceptive, and although today's low-dose OCPs are generally safe and well tolerated, they are not without side effects in all women. Let's explore some possible side effects:

1. Weight Gain

Some women are definitely susceptible to this, particularly those who are always battling with their weight. OCPs containing the more masculine (androgenic) progestogens, may stimulate the appetite and increase the accumulation of body fat, especially in the upper part of the body and the abdomen. Pills containing a high dose of oestrogen may cause fluid retention and weight gain around the hips and thighs. High doses of oestrogen may be associated with an aggravation of varicose veins, leg cramps or aching legs.

2. Nausea and/or Vomiting

This is similar to the 'morning sickness' of pregnancy and is due to the effect of the pill's hormones upon the liver and stomach. Thankfully, it is often temporary. If you have gall bladder disease or gall stones, the OCP often aggravates these problems causing nausea and abdominal pains. The risk of liver tumours (which are rare) is slightly increased in women, who take the combined OCP for a prolonged period.

3. Breakthrough Bleeding

This is defined as bleeding while you are taking the OCP and occurs apart from your regular withdrawal bleed. Because it is usually unpredictable, it is a real nuisance. Breakthrough bleeding may be prevented by changing to a higher dose pill and/or making sure that you take your OCP at the same time every day. Breakthrough bleeding may be a signal that your OCP is not being properly absorbed from your intestines, which may occur if you have an intestinal upset or infection, or if you are on other medication (eg antibiotics, anti-epileptic drugs or asthma medication). Please check with your doctor if breakthrough bleeding keeps occurring, as adequate contraception may not be ensured.

4. Pigmentation of the Skin

The OCP and also pregnancy may induce brown patches of pigmentation, especially on the face and this is called chloasma or the 'mask of pregnancy'. Although this generally fades after the OCP is discontinued, some of the pigmentation may be permanent.

5. Absence of Menstruation (Amenorrhoea)

Around one in every hundred women on the combined OCP fails to menstruate for more than 12 months, after stopping the pill. Such women usually have pre-existing hormonal problems, such as high prolactin levels, weight loss or the Polycystic Ovarian Syndrome. (see page 153) The use of natural progesterone cream will often restore the normal menstrual cycle in these cases. If required their menstrual cycle can be stimulated with more potent hormonal therapy, thus restoring their fertility. In less than 10% of cases of post-pill amenorrhoea, there is no explanation other than the OCP. In such cases it may take up to two years to restore normal fertility, however the use of natural progesterone usually shortens this. The OCP does not exert any significant long-term negative effects on fertility.

6. Mood Changes

The effect of the OCP upon a woman's mental and emotional state is variable. Some find that the OCP increases wellbeing and equanimity by preventing hormonal highs and lows, whereas others find it induces depression and irritability. The latter effect probably arises because the OCP reduces the amount of the brain chemical serotonin that exerts a balancing effect upon moods, mental drive, appetite and sexual desire. In a minority of women, the OCP induces severe and unpleasant mood changes that necessitate its discontinuation. Thankfully, the mood disorders go quickly after stopping the OCP.

7. Loss of sex drive

It is not uncommon for women taking the combined OCP to find that their sex drive (libido) gradually decreases. Although this varies considerably, the reduction in the desire and enjoyment of sex can be quite severe. This is because the OCP induces the liver to make extra amounts of the protein called Sex Hormone Binding Globulin (SHBG). SHBG binds the sex hormones including the naturally produced male hormones, and thus the level of free hormones reduces. The free hormones are the active hormones in the body; less active hormones means less sex drive and less enjoyment of sex. It can take about 6 to 8 weeks after discontinuing the OCP before the high levels of SHBG diminish to normal, when the libido should bounce back to normal levels.

8. Headaches

Headaches, especially of the migrainous type, may be aggravated or brought on for the first time by the combined OCP. If severe migraine occurs, especially if it is associated with visual or neurological disturbance (eg blindness, flashing lights, weakness or numbness of body parts, speech disturbance, etc) the OCP must be stopped immediately. Otherwise there is a much higher risk of stroke occurring.

9. Disorders of the Circulation

The high dose OCPs of the 1960s and early 1970s were associated with an increased risk of cardiovascular disorders, such as high blood pressure, blood clots, heart attacks and strokes. These risks have been greatly reduced with the use of much lower doses of synthetic hormones in today's modern OCPs. They are mainly confined to women over 35, who smoke or have pre-existing cardiovascular risk factors, such as high blood pressure, hardening of the arteries or diabetes. Blood clots are the most common serious side effect of the combined OCP.

Modern low dose combined OCPs can be considered safe but only in 'safe women', as they can be dangerous in 'dangerous women'. Dangerous women are smokers, diabetics, those with high blood pressure, obesity, blood clots, high cholesterol or a previous or family history of heart attacks, angina and strokes.

Smoking is a far greater risk factor for heart disease than the combined OCP. Women over the age of 35, who are on the combined OCP and smoke, should either give up the pill or stop smoking. I believe that any woman, who smokes, regardless of her age, should not take the combined OCP because of the combined harmful effects of the OCP and smoking upon the blood vessels.

Safe women are those who do not have any of the risk factors characterising dangerous women and, according to the Fertility and Maternal Health Drugs Advisory Committee of the Federal Drug Administration, safe women may continue to take a low dose combined OCP up to any age and, if desired, up until the menopause. Even so, safe women over the age of 40, who take the combined OCP, may slightly increase their risk of cardiovascular disease, and if this is found unacceptable, the mini pill (POP) is a good alternative.

The synthetic hormones in the pill tend to increase the level of the blood fats (cholesterol and triglycerides) but these increases are usually slight and not outside of normal limits. You can have your fasting blood fats measured before starting the OCP and again after six months of taking the OCP to detect any adverse changes.

Ideally, all women should have their blood pressure checked three months after starting the OCP to make sure that any increase is not excessive.

Women on the combined OCP, who have major surgery, are much more likely to get post-operative blood clots. So, if you are scheduled for planned surgery, you should be taken off the combined OCP four to six weeks prior to the surgery. Emergency surgery should be preceded by drug therapy to prevent blood clots.

Overall, if you have any cardiovascular risk factors, the combined OCP acts to multiply them. The lower the dose of hormones in the OCP, the safer it is and you should work with your doctor to find the lowest dose OCP that works for you.

Choice of the OCP

Before the OCP is prescribed it is important to take a detailed medical history and do a thorough physical examination. Women who have no risk factors for blood clots can be prescribed any combined OCP containing 35mcg or less of ethinyloestradiol. Women with a past history of blood clots should never take the combined OCP. If there is a family history of blood clots the patient should have blood tests to check their tendency to form blood clots. If these tests show an increased tendency to form blood clots the combined OCP should not be prescribed. In non smoking women over the age of 40, and especially if they are overweight, a low dose combined OCP containing only 20mcg of ethinyloestradiol is safer. In adolescent women who have only been menstruating for several years, the OCP can be prescribed if contraception is needed, as the combined OCP has not been shown to stunt growth or impair future fertility.

In general the lowest dose OCP which allows good control of the monthly cycle should be prescribed, as this will cause less metabolic changes, lower risks and less side effects.

Women who should Not take the Combined OCP

There are certain conditions that preclude you from taking the combined OCP. These are

1. Oestrogen-sensitive cancers, such as uterine or breast cancer. The cause of unexplained vaginal bleeding should be diagnosed before beginning any OCP.
2. Active liver disease or liver tumours.
3. Severe or frequent migraine headaches.
4. Some medical conditions, such as porphyria or diabetes (with circulatory problems)
5. Cardiovascular diseases, such as blood clots, heart disease, strokes,

very high blood pressure, very high cholesterol and triglycerides.

6. Pregnancy.
7. Women over 35 years of age, who smoke cigarettes
8. Women with prolonged immobilisation

The risk of the combined OCP causing blood clots is increased by the following factors

- In cancer patients
- Long distance travel (especially long International jet flights)
- Prolonged immobilisation
- Obesity
- After surgery or trauma
- Kidney or liver disease
- Auto-immune diseases

The Morning-after pill – emergency contraception

From the 1st January 2004 the morning-after pill called "Postinor 2" became available from pharmacies in Australia with out a prescription. This decision was made to allow easier access to emergency contraception to reduce the burden of unwanted pregnancies from rape, sexual assault or unplanned sexual intercourse. It can also be used where a contraceptive method is deemed unreliable.

Postinor 2 tablets contain 750mcg of the synthetic progestogen called lev-onorgestrel.

How does Postinor 2 work?

It may work in several ways

- Preventing sperm from fertilising an egg your ovary has released
- Stopping your ovary from releasing an egg
- Stopping a fertilised egg from attaching itself to the lining of your uterus (womb)

Thus Postinor 2 works to prevent a pregnancy before it is established.

Postinor 2 will not work if you are already pregnant.

How do you use Postinor 2 tablets?

You must take the first tablet within 72 hours (3 days) of having sexual intercourse. Postinor 2 tablets are more effective if they are taken as soon as possible after sex. You must take a second tablet of Postinor 2 twelve (12) hours (and no later than 16 hours) after the first Postinor 2 tablet. You should only use Postinor 2 as an emergency contraceptive. It is not a regular method of contraception and if it is overused it will upset your menstrual cycle.

How effective is Postinor 2?

Postinor 2 prevents around 85% to 97% of expected pregnancies, which is most worthwhile, although it cannot give you a 100% guarantee. Postinor 2 tablets will not protect you against sexually transmitted disease and condoms are your best protection against this.

Side effects of Postinor 2

- Nausea or vomiting
- Spotting or irregular bleeding until your next period is due
- Your next period may be different – it may come earlier or later than expected
- Headaches, abdominal cramps, diarrhoea, fatigue or breast tenderness – these should pass after a few days

Postinor 2 should not be taken if-

You are already pregnant
Your period is late
Since your last menstrual period, you have had unprotected sex more than 72 hours (3 days) ago

Postinor 2 is only available from your pharmacy and you should make sure that you get the correct information about this medication from the pharmacy before you take it.

If you have certain medical problems such as-

Diseases of the small intestines, high blood pressure and/or heart disease, blood clots, diabetes, severe liver disease or breast cancer

then Postinor 2 may not be suitable for you to take as an emergency contraceptive – check with your doctor, family planning clinic or pharmacist first if you have a medical problem.

See your doctor if

You fall pregnant after taking Postinor 2 – there is no evidence that Postinor will harm the developing baby but your doctor may want to check that you do not have an ectopic pregnancy

If you vomit up the tablets

If your expected period is more than 5 days late or is very heavy or painful

Contraceptive Hormone Implants

Contraceptive implants are small plastic rods inserted through the skin into the subcutaneous layer of the upper arm. The insertion technique is a minor surgical procedure (that takes 2.5 minutes) and so is the removal of the rod (takes 1 minute). The implant can be removed at any time at the woman's request but must be removed after 3 years. Doctors should be properly trained in the insertion and removal technique. They are becoming a popular method of contraception with 9 million women in the United States choosing this type of contraception.

The first implant on the market was Norplant which contained the progestogen levonorgestrel. This was taken off the market, as it was found that certain batches of the rods were found to contain less progestogen than others. The newer implants contain different types of progestogens and are easier to insert and remove. The best known of these newer contraceptive implants is Implanon, which is a single rod containing the progestogen called etonogestrel, which is secreted from the rod at a constant rate over a 3 year period, but may provide protection for up to 5 years.

Implanon is designed to provide a more stable release of hormone than Norplant. Etonogestrel is a metabolite of the synthetic progestogen called desogestrel, which means it has less masculine (androgenic) and more progestogenic activity than levonorgestrel. This makes it a better choice for women that have problems with excess androgens including excess facial and body hair, acne and Polycystic Ovarian Syndrome. Implanon is a very effective and convenient contraceptive with failure rates of less then 1%. Steady release of the hormone from the implant into the blood stream avoids the hormone going directly through the liver.

Implanon prevents ovulation by suppressing the pituitary release of luteinising hormone. Implanon does not completely suppress the natural ovarian production of oestrogen, and enough oestrogen continues to be produced from the ovaries to protect the bones from mineral loss. After the implant is removed fertility returns rapidly with 94% of women ovulating within one month after removal.

In breast feeding women Implanon appears to cause no changes to the quality or quantity of the breast milk. The growth of the baby is not affected although a small amount of etonogestrel is detected in the breast milk. Thus a lactating woman needs to discuss these issues with her doctor. Generally speaking women who suffer with period pains find that Implanon reduces their pain.

Oral Contraceptive Pill Side Effects and their Remedies Chart

SIDE EFFECT	AVOID	USE	OTHER MEASURES
Weight gain	High dose OCPs	Mini pill (POP) Triphasic pills	Regular exercise Low-carbohydrate diet Eat plenty of vegetables and fruits
Nausea, Vomiting	High dose OCPs	Mini pill (POP) Triphasic pills may be better tolerated Progestogen hormone implant	Take OCP with food and a good multi-vitamin Liver tonics may help Have a check of your gall bladder & liver
Breakthrough bleeding	Mini pill (POP) Low-dose OCPs	Higher dose pills or tailor-made OCP from your doctor. OCPs containing the progestogen norethisterone reduce breakthrough bleeding	Take the OCP at the *same time* each day. See your doctor for a gynaecological examination.
Facial Pigmentation (chloasma)	Combined OCPs	Mini pill (POP)	Sunscreen lotion Broad brim hat Depigmentation cream at night Liver tonics help to fade the pigmentation
Breast tenderness	High dose OCPs	Mini pill (POP) Triphasic OCPs Progestogen hormone implant	Evening Primrose & Flaxseed Oil Selenium & vitamin B Have a breast examination
Mood disorders Poor libido	High dose OCPs Cyproterone acetate (Androcur)	Mini pill (POP) Choose OCPs that contain the "friendly" progestogens desogestrel or gestodene	Flaxseed oil Power Woman multi vitamin-mineral Hypericum (St John's Wort)
Headaches Migraines	All combined OCPs	Mini-pill (POP) Progestogen hormone implant	Increase water intake. Raw juicing Magnesium Complete (2 tablets twice daily) Liver tonic capsules See your doctor for a check up
High blood pressure Blood clots	All combined OCPs	Mini pill (POP) Progestogen hormone implant	Vitamin C, garlic, Magnesium tablets 2 litres water daily Raw vegetable juices
Vaginal candida	High dose OCPs	Triphasic OCPs or mini pill (POP) Progestogen hormone implant	Follow a low carb diet Avoid sugar & alcohol Take Olive leaf extract, selenium, zinc & acidophilus Tea tree oil vaginal douche gel

Possible side effects on Implanon are

- Weight gain – studies have shown an increase of 2.6% in body weight over a 2 year period of Implanon use. In susceptible women etonogestrel will increase Syndrome X and blood sugar levels and thus it must be used with caution in diabetics
- Pimples and acne are generally improved but some women will notice an increase
- Breast tenderness
- Mood disorders
- A change in menstrual bleeding patterns - irregular bleeding is not uncommon, and in 10% of users this can be heavy and prolonged, which requires removal of the rod.

The body's hormone levels rapidly return to normal after the rod is removed and usually a normal period will occur within 2 months after removal.

Implanon may cause the development of small cysts on the ovaries due to follicular activity with no ovulation however these cysts generally cause no symptoms and resolve spontaneously.

Contraceptive Injections – Depo-Provera

The Depo-Provera injection contains the progestogen called medroxy-progesterone acetate and has been used world-wide as a contraceptive for many years. For years there were concerns about the long term safety of Depo-Provera and it was not until 1994 that it was licensed in Australia for contraceptive use.

Depo-Provera is given as an intramuscular injection every 12 weeks and contains 150mg of medroxy-progesterone acetate. Depo-Provera is a very reliable method of contraception with failure rates of less than 1%.

Depo-Provera injections will always cause the menstrual cycle to change – irregular bleeding is common during the first few months after the injection is given, and then most women will find that their periods disappear or that only very light irregular bleeding occurs especially with prolonged use. Indeed after 12 months of use, 80% of women have no periods (amenorrhoea) or occasional spotting only. This reduction in bleeding can be a welcome relief for women plagued with heavy or painful periods.

Depo-Provera is a useful contraceptive for

- Women who cannot remember to take a pill everyday
- Women who have medical problems that make them unable to take oestrogen
- As a method of contraception in breast feeding women, as it does not affect the quality/quantity of breast milk
- In women with epilepsy, as its effectiveness is not reduced by anti-convulsant drugs

Possible side effects of Depo-Provera

Weight gain

Acne

Moodiness

A possible decrease in bone density with long term use, however this is considered controversial, and is generally considered insignificant in women using Depo-Provera for less than 5 years. Studies show that the bone density quickly returns to normal after ceasing Depo-Provera injections.

A delay in the return to normal fertility after ceasing use of Depo-Provera – it often takes several months, and occasionally longer, before regular menstrual cycles resume

If side effects do occur, it is necessary to wait for 3 months until the injection wears off.

Contraceptive Patch – OrthoEvra

This is the first patch that has been approved for use as a contraceptive. The patch is applied once a week, for three weeks, and then left off for one week. A withdrawal bleed will occur during the patch-free week. The contraceptive efficiency of the patch is similar to the pill and is 99% effective. Women using the contraceptive patch report similar side effects to those of the OCP with the addition of irritation at site of application. In clinical trials the patch appeared to be a less effective contraceptive in women who weighed more than 90kgs. The patch contains a combination of the hormones ethinyl oestradiol and norelgestromin (a synthetic progestogen). The progestogen norelgestromin has shown minimal masculinising (androgenic) effects in the trials of the patch.

The patch will deliver an effective dose of the hormones regardless of the application site. As with any hormonal therapy, the patch should not be applied to the breasts.

Benefits of the contraceptive patch include-

It supplies an effective dose of hormones into the blood stream under conditions of heat, humidity and immersion in water. Thus active women can wear the patch while exercising or swimming.

It delivers a steady dose of hormones into the blood stream avoiding highs and lows that can occur through oral dosing - this may be particularly beneficial for women who suffer from migraines triggered by a drop in oestrogen levels.

It avoids 'first pass' metabolism of the hormones by the liver, taking excess workload off this important organ. This is because the method of delivery is via the skin into the blood stream (transdermal absorption)

Its success does not depend upon a good memory - as the patch is applied for 7 days straight, women do not need to remember to take a daily pill, making it better for the forgetful among us!

Intra-uterine devices - Mirena

Intra-uterine devices (IUDs) are an increasingly popular method of contraception worldwide. Mirena is an IUD that contains the hormone levonorgestrel, which is slowly released from the IUD. Mirena is approved for up to 5 years of use in the United States. The failure rate is less than 0.3%.

IUD's should not be used in women with a history of pelvic inflammatory disease or lower genital tract infection. Mirena does not seem to cause the heavy menstrual bleeding that older types of IUD's were known to do and because it contains a progestogen will tend to reduce heavy bleeding. As with all IUD's, Mirena is associated with a higher risk of ectopic pregnancy.

Contraception in the Future

No one has yet found the ideal hormone contraceptive although we are getting close.

In particular, experts agree that it is best to use the smallest dose of synthetic hormones and also to use a progesterone that is 'friendly' to our blood fats and cardiovascular system. These friendly progesterones are non-masculine (non-androgenic) and are also friendly to our skin, as they are more feminine and help to control acne and facial hair. Examples of these friendly feminine progesterones are cyproterone acetate, desogestrel, drosperinone and gestodene.

In Europe, Australia and New Zealand, women have access to OCPs containing small doses (20mcg as opposed to 30mcg) of oestrogen combined with friendly progesterones such as desogestrel, gestodene and norgestimate. Brand names of these pills are Mercilon, Minulet Marvelon, Femoden and Trioden. These are ideal OCPs for older women or indeed for the majority of women.

Contraceptive implants and patches are an important option for women who cannot take combined oral contraceptive pills. These will include women with diabetes mellitus, vascular disease, high cholesterol/triglycerides, and/or a history of stroke and heart disease, migraines and depression, or smokers over 35 years of age.

CHAPTER 9

Surgical Sterilisation may be more than you bargained for

Surgical sterilisation in a woman is known as tubal ligation and most women relate to this as "having their tubes tied". This is a surgical procedure that interrupts or blocks the fallopian tube of the uterus. This prevents the egg from meeting with the sperm so that fertilisation, which normally occurs inside the fallopian tube, cannot occur. (see Diagram 11)

After tubal ligation the tiny egg continues to be released every month from the ovary and is broken down and absorbed into the body. Tubal ligation is a permanent form of sterilisation and no one should have this procedure done unless they are absolutely certain that they do not want any more children. Surgical reversal of a tubal ligation can be attempted but it does not always succeed. Micro surgical reversal of tubal ligation can give pregnancy rates as high as 70% but a 100% guarantee can never be given and so at the outset, it should be considered irreversible. Even if the fallopian tubes can be rejoined with micro surgery, it is often impossible to rejoin the ovarian blood vessels that may have been divided or damaged at tubal ligation. Pregnancy following reversal of tubal ligation may be associated with hormonal imbalances and miscarriage and may require hormonal therapy.

Tubal ligation is a very commonly performed operation – with approximately 650,000 American and 50,000 Australian women undergoing it every year.

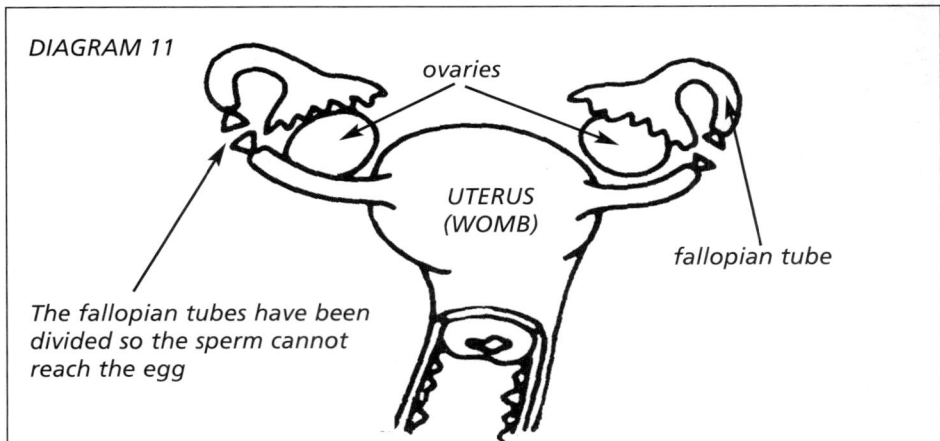

DIAGRAM 11

ovaries

UTERUS
(WOMB)

fallopian tube

The fallopian tubes have been divided so the sperm cannot reach the egg

It is often taken very casually with many women believing it is the easiest thing to do, once their family is complete. Indeed, having your 'tubes tied' seems so simple – no more pills or messy diaphragms to remember, just one day in hospital and you're on your way free of the worry of unwanted pregnancy. However, it is not always hassle-free and without side effects, as you will soon see, and it is a pity that women undergoing tubal ligation are not always advised of all its possible long-term effects.

How effective is a tubal ligation?

There is no doubt that tubal ligation is effective contraception, as the failure rate is very low with three pregnancies in every 1,000 sterilised women. Said another way tubal ligation is 99.5% effective as a method of permanent birth control. Tubal ligation provides effective contraception immediately after the operation

Techniques of Tubal Ligation

The fallopian tubes may be blocked by different methods, such as cutting and tying them off (Pomeroy technique), burning with an electric current or clipping them with metal or plastic rings or clips. Tubal ligation is done through a laparoscope (medical telescope) with key-hole surgery or through a very small lower abdominal incision (mini-laparotomy). Tubal ligation is usually done under a general anaesthetic.

It is important that you check which method your surgeon will use, as each method has different risks and complications associated with it.

1. The technique of burning the tubes (tubal diathermy) is now outmoded and should not be done, as it is associated with a high chance of causing damage to the surrounding blood vessels, organs and intestines and the formation of scar tissue. It has a higher failure rate than clipping the tubes and is more likely to cause heavy menstrual periods in the future.

2. Cutting or tying the tubes (Pomeroy technique) has been used for many years and was most commonly done after childbirth. It has several disadvantages – it has a higher failure rate than clipping the tubes; the area of damage to the tubes and surrounding blood vessels is higher than clipping with more chance of damaging the blood supply to the ovary. If it is performed immediately after childbirth, it is a tragedy if anything goes wrong with the baby and it subsequently dies, as the Pomeroy technique is not easily reversed.

3. If you are absolutely sure that you want a tubal ligation, the best method to ask for is clipping the tubes, which can be done through a

laparoscope (long narrow telescope) that is inserted into the abdominal cavity through a one-centimetre incision. The abdominal cavity is filled with carbon dioxide gas, which allows the surgeon to see the organs more clearly. The laparoscope uses fiberoptics and functions like a hollow flashlight, so that the surgeon can see your organs and insert surgical tools through the hollow bore of the laparoscope. The tubes are compressed with a silastic ring (Falope ring) or metal clips (Filschie clips). The falope ring acts like a rubber band on the tubes and the filschie clip acts like a metal staple and clamps the tubes closed. In the hands of a good and experienced surgeon, clipping of the tubes is less likely to cause damage to the surrounding blood vessels that supply the ovary and should be less likely to result in long-term problems with the function of the ovaries. Clipping the tubes causes damage to a much smaller area of the tubes than either the burning or tying techniques and so is more easily reversed if you should change your mind. The falope rings and filschie clips are the safest technique with less risk of complications post-operatively.

Post-operative problems after tubal ligation, such as haemorrhage, bowel damage, infections, peritonitis, blood clots, damage to surrounding organs and severe post-operative pain occur in 3% to 5% of cases. However, surgeons experienced in the technique of clipping the tubes tell me that this method has less than a 1% chance of such complications.

Currently, with all available methods of tubal ligation, there exists a small chance (which varies between the methods used) of damaging the blood supply to the ovary, as the ovarian blood vessels run alongside the fallopian tubes on their way to the ovary. (see Diagram 12 page 108). It is easy to see how these blood vessels could be compressed or cut during surgery to the closely adjacent tube.

Researchers in Australia have shown that blocking the blood supply to the ovarian artery can result in high blood pressure in the ovary, which could result in the tissues of the ovary being damaged. If this occurs, the ovary may not function normally and its production of the sex hormones oestrogen and progesterone, which depends upon adequate blood and oxygen supply, may be reduced (Ref 26,28). More precise micro surgical techniques of tubal ligation, with careful conservation of the ovarian blood supply would provide a less hit and miss approach to the chances of long-term problems with ovarian function.

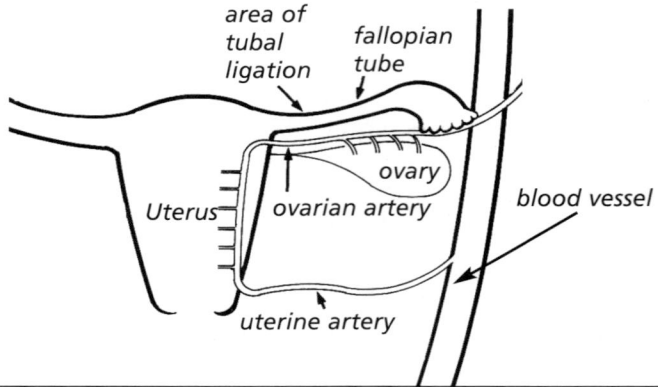

DIAGRAM 12
Blood supply to ovary and uterus

area of tubal ligation

fallopian tube

ovary

blood vessel

Uterus

ovarian artery

uterine artery

What are the possible problems after tubal ligation?

1. Menstrual and Gynaecological Problems

Since 1951, there have been reports in the literature that women have a higher risk of heavy menstrual bleeding, irregular bleeding and hysterectomy after tubal ligation. The incidence of pelvic pain, period pains, longer periods and pain during sexual intercourse may also be higher. Endometriosis may also be more likely after surgical sterilisation. These problems often get worse with increasing time after the tubal ligation. Another irony of tubal ligation is that it may increase your chance of needing a hysterectomy in the future, although many women believe that it will provide an end to their contraceptive and gynaecological problems. (Ref 23-29).

A study in the USA followed up 200 women after tubal ligation. At least 16.5% of these women developed abnormal bleeding requiring a hysterectomy within ten years of sterilisation, which was three times more than the hysterectomy rate in non-sterilised women. A Scottish study found that the hysterectomy rate after tubal ligation was 9.3% compared to 2.5% in non-sterilised women.

Many surgeons minimise these complications refusing to admit that they have any relationship with tubal ligation. They often ascribe them to the fact that the patient is getting older, has come off the oral contraceptive pill since sterilisation, and would have developed these problems anyway. Therefore, it is difficult to determine the true incidence of subsequent gynaecological problems linked to tubal ligation. If tubal ligation fails and pregnancy occurs, then there is a greater possibility of this being a tubal or ectopic pregnancy.

2. Hormonal Problems

Some researchers believe that hormonal deficiencies and imbalances may affect up to 60% of women after tubal ligation and this area urgently needs more scientific scrutiny. Some women do escape any significant hormonal problems after tubal ligation, while others experience symptoms due to oestrogen deficiency or imbalances of oestrogen and progesterone.(Ref 26,28)

The chances of developing hormonal problems depend upon damage to the ovarian blood supply and this depends upon the skill and technique of the surgeon. The production of oestrogen from the ovary is more likely to be affected than is the production of progesterone, as oestrogen needs more oxygen for the many steps necessary in its synthesis by the ovary. If the ovarian blood supply is reduced by tubal ligation, the supply of oxygen to the ovary is diminished, resulting in inadequate oestrogen synthesis.

Women with inadequate amounts of oestrogen in their body will typically complain of the following symptoms

- Loss of libido (interest in sex)
- Reduced orgasms
- Hot flushes
- Reduction in breast size
- Vaginal dryness & discomfort
- Discomfort during sexual intercourse
- Bladder problems
- A possible increase in musculo-skeletal aches and pains (fibromyalgia)
- Possible reduction in the quality of sleep

Because oestrogen is involved in the maintenance of collagen, women with low oestrogen levels may complain of more rapid ageing of the skin and aches and pains, as collagen is lost from the skin and bones. (Refer to the Oestrogen Level Score Chart on Page 110 to see if you are lacking in oestrogen). Women lacking both oestrogen and progesterone usually complain of mood disorders, fatigue, pre-menstrual syndrome and menstrual disturbances. Understandably, women with these hormonal problems are at greater risk of marital and family discord. The development of such hormonal problems can be gradual and insidious, especially if not recognised for what they are, and may take several years after tubal ligation to fully develop. I have seen many women with such problems, who were searching for an answer.

OESTROGEN DEFICIENCY SYNDROME	SCORE(0-3)
Depression and mood changes	
Anxiety and/or irritability	
Unloved or unwanted feelings	
Poor memory and concentration	
Poor sleeping patterns (insomnia)	
Fatigue	
Reduction in orgasms	
Joint pains, back ache, increase in arthritis	
Muscle pains (fibromyalgia)	
New facial hair	
Dry skin and/or sudden wrinkling	
Crawling, itching, burning sensations in the skin	
Reduced sexual desire	
Frequency or burning of urination	
Discomfort during sexual intercourse	
Vaginal dryness	
Hot flushes and/or excessive sweating	
Light-headedness or dizziness	
Increase in headaches	
YOUR TOTAL SCORE	

This chart is derived from Professor Nordin's Menopause Questionnaire, Institute of Medical and Veterinary Science, Adelaide, South Australia.

The symptoms that are characteristic of oestrogen deficiency may be grouped together in the chart above and scored according to the following scale:

Absent = 0   Mild = 1   Moderate = 2   Severe = 3

If your score for all these symptoms is 15 or more, then it is likely that you are suffering with a deficiency of oestrogen. If your score is around 30, your body is crying out for oestrogen. Oestrogen deficiency can be confirmed or refuted with a simple blood test to check your level of oestrogen and Follicle Stimulating Hormone (FSH). If there is a deficiency of oestrogen, your FSH level will be over 20, and often higher.

It is an interesting exercise to score your symptoms of oestrogen deficiency before and after commencing Hormone Replacement Therapy (HRT).

The Story of Virginia

Virginia was a prolific writer of children's stories and she was finding it more and more difficult to use her computer because of pain in her neck, forearms and wrists. Shopping and picking up her two young children were also proving stressful, as she had lower back pain, which restricted her bending over. She felt rather cheated and angry, as she was only 39 and was suffering with symptoms that she thought were typical of a woman much older. She was not used to this, as she had previously been very sportive and fit.

It had all started one year after her tubal ligation, which had been performed immediately after the caesarean section required for the birth of her last child. She became increasingly exhausted, which was due to undiagnosed anaemia due to her heavy painful period that had developed in the last six months. Her beautiful athletic physique had also changed and she had developed lumpy cellulite around her abdomen, although she was following a very healthy low carbohydrate diet. She found that her skin looked thinner and dry and started to age more rapidly.

Virginia's creativity also seemed to be flagging and the magical stories did not flow from her brain with the same ease and colour. She could not understand why she felt so down, as she was trying to do all the right things and even her supplements of vitamins and minerals did not give her a lift.

Fortunately, Virginia's doctor had the foresight to refer her to a hormone specialist, as he remembered how different she had been several years ago and he suspected she had a hormonal problem. The specialist ordered blood tests, which showed that Virginia had subnormal levels of oestrogen and progesterone, and looked as though she was going to have an early menopause. She was in the pre-menopause, as her FSH levels were still under 20, and she still had regular menstrual periods. Virginia's blood tests also revealed severe iron deficiency anaemia for which she was given iron supplements. For her hormonal imbalance she was given a troche (lozenge) containing natural oestradiol 1mg, and natural progesterone 100mg, combined in one troche. She was instructed to take half a troche twice daily.

Within six weeks, Virginia felt her aches ad pains disappear and her mental and emotional state improved. Once again, she was churning out her children's stories and felt like playing with her children. She was delighted to find the lumpy cellulite reducing without having to starve herself to death and she now had the energy to resume her aerobics classes at the gym.

Virginia still felt a little cheated, as her gynaecologist had not warned her that tubal ligation can result in hormonal problems and she felt that she was rather young to start Hormone Replacement Therapy. Had she known, she would never have had her tubes tied.

At least her symptoms had been recognised for what they were or else she feared that she may have continued to age rapidly and needed anti-inflammatory drugs. Virginia was amazed that the hormones oestrogen and progesterone exerted such a powerful influence in her body, as she had never before been a victim of her hormones.

Can hormone problems after tubal ligation be treated effectively?

In a significant number of women with "hormonal problems" after tubal ligation, a hormonal state similar to the pre-menopause is found. This means that the hormonal output from the ovaries is reduced to a level that we find typically in a woman in her mid to late 40s, who is approaching the menopause.

To assess the level of oestrogen and progesterone production by your ovaries, you can ask your doctor to measure the amount of these hormones and also the pituitary hormone FSH in blood tests. Salivary tests for progesterone are also helpful (see page 178)

You have a right to know your hormone levels, as it is vitally important because long-term consequences of oestrogen and progesterone deficiency could be an increased risk of cardiovascular disease, osteoporosis, premature ageing or cancer.

Once your doctor has proven that you have a hormonal deficiency or imbalance, this can be treated with Hormone Replacement Therapy using natural bio-identical hormones. This can be tailor made to suit your hormonal imbalance and the smallest effective dose can be found over a period of 6 months. I personally prefer to use the hormone creams as I find that they are less potent and have less tendency to produce break through bleeding. Also if any side effects occur it is so simple to reduce the dosage. I recommend that you have 6-monthly blood tests to check the level of your hormones whilst on any form of HRT, so as to avoid using excess doses, which could lead to a build up of hormones in the blood and tissues.

Long term Hormone Replacement Therapy remains controversial because of its association with an increased risk of breast cancer and some women choose to discontinue it after 12 months. However if symptoms recur and your quality of life becomes poor, you will need to work with your doctor to find the lowest dose of natural bio-identical hormones that will relieve your symptoms. Let's face it – who want's to live to 100 feeling like a dried up old prune !!

Oestrogen replacement can also be given in the form of an oestrogen patch, which is a sticky transparent membrane impregnated with natural oestrogen. Some patches also contain synthetic progesterone with the oestrogen. The patch is applied to the skin of the buttock, abdomen or trunk (excluding the breast) and releases oestrogen through the skin, which absorbs into your bloodstream.

Although I rarely use oestrogen implants in my patients, I will discuss them here, as some doctors still use them and some women still ask for them. The implants consist of small pellets of pure crystalline oestradiol and resemble a tiny piece of spaghetti. They come in various strengths to suit individual needs and are somewhat expensive, although the cost can be claimed from most private health funds. They can be painlessly implanted into the fatty layer of your abdomen or buttocks under a local anaesthetic and many doctors use a small hollow tube with a sharp cutting edge to slide the pellet neatly into your fat.

Depending upon the strength of the implant chosen by your doctor, an implant will continue to release oestrogen directly into your blood stream for between four to twelve months, which is ideal for those who cannot remember to take tablets.

Of all the types of HRT, an implant comes closest to copying the function of your own ovaries as in both cases oestrogen is released directly into the bloodstream and carried to the various oestrogen-dependent tissues of your body. Thus, your hungry cells get their supply of oestrogen before the liver enzymes can break it down. Unfortunately, this is not so with oestrogen tablets, which are first broken down by passage through the liver after their absorption from the gut. Thus, the liver could be said to weaken the effect of oestrogen tablets upon your cells, whereas the oestrogen implant is able to deliver a direct supply of oestrogen. For the same reason the implants are very potent and I have found very high levels of oestrogen in blood tests in many of my patients who used the implants. These high levels can reach up to 4000 or more, and I find this worrying, and thus I do not recommend the use of implants for the long term. Now that we have the patches and even better the creams containing natural hormones, we do not have to overdose our selves with oestrogen.

Today HRT has become very versatile and different combinations of natural progesterone and oestrogen patches, implants and creams can be tried with your own doctor until you find the programme that suits your individual mental, physical and sexual requirements. If you require more information on doctors who do this type of HRT call the Women's Health Advisory Service on 0246 558855 or visit www.whas.com.au

If you still have a uterus, oestrogen replacement must be accompanied by some form of progesterone, whether it be natural or synthetic. This is because oestrogen given alone will increase the risk of uterine cancer. Synthetic progesterone is usually given in tablet form and must be given for twelve to fourteen days of every calendar month to balance the oestrogen and regulate your cycle to bring on a regular menstrual bleed.

If your periods are very heavy and/or painful, you may benefit much more by taking progesterone alone. This can be a choice of synthetic or natural progesterone although the majority of women find that the natural progesterone is much more pleasant to take. This is because the natural progesterone not only reduces heavy painful periods but also increases well being and enhances a happy stable state of mind.

Some doctors use the oral contraceptive pill (OCP) routinely to treat all women with "hormonal problems" after tubal ligation. This may work for some, however as contraception is no longer required, and the OCP contains synthetic hormones with possible side effects, I believe that there are much better options.

The Story of Ruth

Ruth looked tired and depressed as she slumped into the chair on the other side of my desk. The most obvious reason for her fatigue was probably that she had five children, all under ten years of age. However, as she related the sequence of her symptom, the jigsaw pieces starting coming together.

Two and a half years ago, Ruth had undergone surgical sterilisation from a surgeon, who had used the outmoded technique of burning the tubes. She had not been told what technique the surgeon would use, as the consent form she had signed did not explore the alternatives. Ruth had thought this was her only way out, as she could not tolerate the oral contraceptive pill and her husband refused vasectomy.

Eighteen months after her sterilisation, she developed heavy painful periods, heralded by increasing pre-menstrual tension with severe mood changes. She felt resentful towards her husband, who could not understand her unpredictable moods and loss of interest in sex. She experienced a constant dull throbbing pain in her pelvis and sexual intercourse was acutely painful on deep penetration.

Ruth was nearly 40 and felt that her hormonal problems may be due to early menopause, especially as she felt she was ageing rapidly. Her rapidly diminishing self esteem and confidence were not helped by her husband, who felt that her symptoms were psychosomatic.

I asked her if she ever felt good. She replied that at the end of seven days of menstrual bleeding, she felt a bit like her old self and said, "That's when I wear high heels again, cook cakes and take the kids out, but I only feel normal for seven days, then the rotten pre-menstrual syndrome takes the wind out of my sails".

Ruth wanted to know if she could have her tubal ligation reversed. I said this was doubtful as her surgeon had used the burning method, which often causes damage to the fragile tubes and the blood supply to the ovaries. Trying to reverse this damage would be no guarantee to cure her hormonal problems and would also involve more surgery and pain.

I encouraged Ruth to try hormonal therapy. Blood and urine tests revealed that Ruth's ovaries were not functioning well, presumably because of damage to their blood supply induced by burning of the tubes and blood vessels at the time of sterilisation.

Ruth started on natural oestrogen tablets (Progynova 1mg twice daily) everyday and progesterone (Provera 5mg) for the first twelve days of every calendar month. The Provera tablets were necessary to balance the oestrogen and regulate her cycle and they would bring on a menstrual period around the twelfth day of every calendar month.

This treatment relieved her pre-menstrual tension, depression, pelvic pain and heavy bleeding and she started to get on top of this again.

Her flagging libido remained a problem so we checked her level of male hormones, which are necessary for a healthy sex drive, orgasmic ability and so called 'feminine virility'. We found that her male hormones were almost non-existent, which explained why she felt asexual, which she described as "almost like a eunuch".

Ruth and I decided that this was best overcome by giving her an injection of natural oestrogen and testosterone every month, with this injection being given at the end of every menstrual period. This was to continue for three months and would build up her body's male hormones to a degree sufficient to increase libido but without causing side effects, such as facial hair or acne. The Primodian injection proved nothing short of a miraculous and Ruth began to feel like a vital, sexual and happy human being for the first time in three years. Once the course of hormone injections was finished I started her on a cream containing natural testosterone.

There are thousands of women like Ruth, who are standing on the sidelines, struggling with their health and waiting for enlightened doctors to draw the curtains on the astounding benefits of natural hormone replacement.

Until more long-term studies of women after tubal ligation are available, we can only guess at the number of women having hysterectomies to relieve their post-sterilisation symptoms. They should be given all the alternatives to hysterectomy and not be told that it is the only answer.

Precautions before having a Tubal Ligation

As has been seen, surgical sterilisation or tubal ligation is not always free of hassles and should not be taken casually. I would not advise my patients to undergo tubal ligation, unless they were aware of possible side effects. Tubal ligation can be ideal if a further pregnancy would be a catastrophe, as in women with severe diabetes, heart, kidney or liver disease. I would advise any woman with gynaecological problems, such as heavy and/or painful periods, fibroids, endometriosis, pelvic pain, pre-menstrual syndrome or a past history of postnatal depression to avoid tubal ligation.

Until surgeons have perfected and standardised surgical techniques (preferably microsurgical) for tubal ligation, I think that younger women considering this operation should think about the possibility that current techniques (which vary widely) may put them at a higher risk for hormonal and gynaecological problems and reduced ovarian function.

Older women may have little to gain from tubal ligation. They already face the likelihood of diminished ovarian function in the pre-menopausal years and tubal ligation will give them less contraceptive time than younger women. Furthermore, they are less fertile anyway, so that simple and safe contraceptive methods, such as the progesterone only pill, diaphragms and vaginal rings and hormone implants are relatively more effective.

If you really want a tubal ligation, make sure that your personal life is stable and happy. I have seen many women, who later wanted a reversal of their tubal ligation. If you are currently taken the oral contraceptive pill and are considering having a tubal ligation, come off the pill for six months before having the operation. If during this six-month break, your periods are heavy or painful, you are not a good candidate for a tubal ligation as this operation may increase these menstrual problems.

Before having a tubal ligation, have a thorough gynaecological examination, pelvic examination and pap smear and, if you have abnormal bleeding, you should have a dilatation and curettage of the uterus. This will exclude the presence of cancer of the uterus or cervix or huge fibroids that may require a hysterectomy in the near future, in which case, a tubal ligation would have been an entirely unnecessary and unpleasant experience.

Finally, I believe that the consent forms for tubal ligation should be expanded to include all the potential complications and problems (including the increased risk of hysterectomy) that may occur in the long term subsequent to this procedure. The consent form should also state that more research is needed to determine the real incidence of these problems. Then we could say that women are really able to give valid informed consent to a surgical procedure that may have a lasting effect upon their lives.

What other methods of female sterilisation are available?

Essure

A relatively new method of permanent birth control is called Essure and involves the insertion of a device into the canal of each of the fallopian tubes. Over time tissue from the tubes grows into the device and blocks

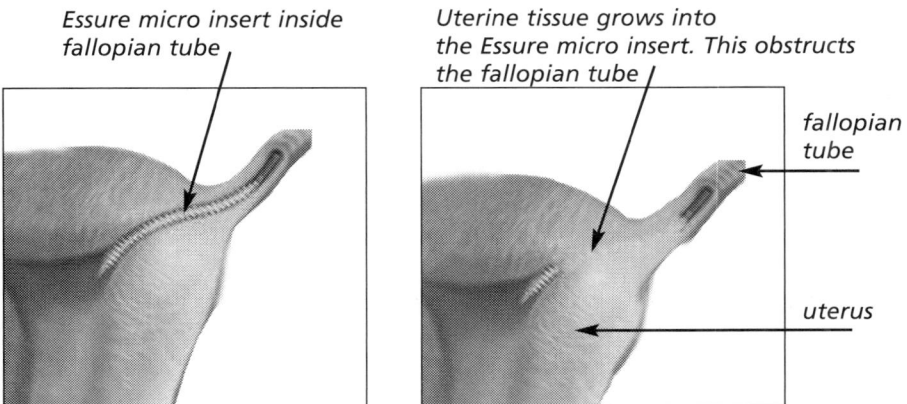

Essure micro insert inside fallopian tube

Uterine tissue grows into the Essure micro insert. This obstructs the fallopian tube

fallopian tube

uterus

the tubes, which prevents the sperm from travelling into the tube to fertilise the egg. The device is known as a micro-insert and consists of a stainless steel inner coil, a nitinol super-elastic outer coil and polyethylene fibres. The micro-insert is 4 centimetres long and 0.8 millimetres in diameter. After insertion the micro-insert remains anchored inside the fallopian tube.

A big advantage of the Essure method of sterilisation is that it can be done without a general anaesthetic and without cutting any skin or organ parts. Thus there is no scar. The Essure insert is inserted into each tube through a small telescope known as a hysteroscope and the procedure takes only 30 minutes. The hysteroscope is inserted through the vagina and cervix into the inside cavity of the uterus to visualise the opening of the fallopian tubes and the insert is accurately fitted into each tube through a narrow tube (catheter).

After the Essure device has been inserted it is necessary to wait 3 months before contraception is reliable. This method of sterilisation is relatively new and research into its reliability and effects is still ongoing. Clinical studies have shown that the contraceptive reliability of Essure after one year is 97%, which means there is a 3% failure rate.

The Essure method of sterilisation may be a better option than tubal ligation, as there is no damage to the blood supply to the ovaries with the Essure method. Thus in women with hormonal imbalances such as heavy menstrual periods, or premenstrual mood disorder the Essure method would be less likely to worsen these problems compared to tubal ligation.

For more information visit www.essure.com

CHAPTER 10

How your hormones affect your appearance

When the body's hormones are out of balance, dramatic and distressing changes in physical appearance and demeanour can take place. Let us look at the most common of these imbalances.

Too Many Male Hormones

Women need a correct balance of male type hormones (androgens) in their bodies in order to function normally on a physical and sexual level.

There are several male hormones, the best known being testosterone but in reality these hormones are just as much female as male; the only difference being that women normally produce much less of them than men. Indeed, male hormones are essential to normal female assertiveness and improve mood and confidence. They can help us to cope with physical and mental stress and can be powerful anti-depressants in both sexes.

The female ovary secretes three important male hormones called testosterone, androstenedione and dehydroepiandrosterone (DHEA). Male hormones are also produced by the adrenal glands, liver, fat and skin. In a woman's normal menstrual cycle, the blood level of male hormones increases at mid-cycle about the time of ovulation and this is why women are most sexy at this time!

For women it is most desirable that a correct balance of male hormones is maintained because if they become excessive, masculine changes can occur in the appearance. Let us take a look at how excessive amounts of male hormones can affect your body hair, scalp hair and skin.

Body Hair

Excessive male hormones can lead to an increase in hair on areas of the body, where hair is normally prominent only in males. You would notice an increase in hair on your chin, upper lip, the sides of your face, chest and lower abdomen and thighs. The hair follicles are sensitive to male hormones and increasing levels of these hormones promote the rate of hair growth and the transformation of fine, soft or 'vellus' hair to coarser 'terminal' hair. This effect occurs in hair on the face and the body but not on the scalp.

The problem of excessive facial and body hair is called hirsutism and it troubles up to 30% of all women in varying degrees, which explains the high frequency of advertisements in women's magazines for centres removing excessive facial and body hair. Most women with hirsutism have only a mild degree and do not have any serious hormonal imbalances, which would lead to irreversible masculinisation.

What Causes Hirsutism?

The most common cause of hirsutism is a slight over-production of male hormones from the ovaries and from the adrenal glands. Excess body fat, especially if it is concentrated in the upper part of the body (the trunk and abdomen) will produce male type hormones and the more overweight you are in this area, the higher the level of male hormones will be. It is interesting to note that fat tissue is hormonally active and can be a significant source of hormone production.

The excess male hormones can be detected in blood tests, and the most sensitive indicator is a test called the Free Androgen Index (FAI) – see page 177. Other blood tests that should be done are total testosterone, free testosterone and DHEA-S levels, which may show abnormally high levels.

The excess male hormones do not cause any ill-effects upon health or fertility, but do stimulate the annoying growth of body hair. In some women with mild hirsutism, blood levels of male hormones are completely normal and the fault lies in excessive sensitivity of their skin and hair follicles to normal levels of male hormones.

There is often a family history of hirsutism in related females and it occurs most commonly in women of Southern European and Middle Eastern descent. Racial and genetic factors are obviously important. Hirsutism is rare among oriental women.

Women, who are overweight, are more likely to suffer with hirsutism because their excessive amounts of fat are associated with higher levels of male hormones. If they lose weight, their levels of male hormones usually decrease with a corresponding reduction in body and facial hair.

The gynaecological disorder of Polycystic Ovarian Syndrome (PCOS) can cause hirsutism. In this condition, the ovaries may develop many small follicle cysts around their periphery.

PCOS is quite common and around one in every six women probably has a tendency to polycystic ovaries. These polycystic ovaries secrete excessive amounts of male hormones, which may result in hirsutism, acne and infrequent menstruation. Many women with polycystic ovaries are over-weight and should try to lose their excessive weight, which may in itself restore regular menstruation and normal levels of male hormones. Conversely, if such women gain weight, their menstrual periods become less frequent and acne and hirsutism increase. In some obese women, it seems that excessive amounts of male hormones produced from their fat somehow 'virilize' their ovaries stimulating them to produce excessive male hormones and this can become a vicious circle. The tendency to poly-cystic ovaries is inherited and may be triggered by stress, weight gain or a high carbohydrate diet.

Some medications may increase body and facial hair such as the anabolic steroids used by athletes and body builders. Other drugs, such as Danazol, Dilantin and some brands of the oral contraceptive pill containing the mas-culine progestogen norgestrel may also increase facial hair.

Hirsutism is generally mild to moderate in degree but if it is severe, or of rapid onset and progression, tests must be done to check for a severe glandular disorder that may lead to extreme masculine changes in appear-ance called virilization.

Virilization

This describes the masculine changes that occur in women with very high levels of male hormones. In such cases, there will be a dramatic and wide-spread increase in facial and body hair, acne, loss of menstruation and shrinkage of the breasts. It is usually frighteningly obvious as, in essence, a woman finds herself transforming into a man. She will notice recession of her scalp hairline with a male pattern of baldness, deepening of her voice, enlargement of her clitoris into a mini-penis and a defeminization of her figure.

Virilization is a rare event and is always associated with a serious hormon-al problem, such as a tumour of the ovaries or adrenal glands. In such cases, these tumours produce large amounts of male hormones and blood tests reveal greatly increased levels of androgens that may be even greater than those found in males. These tumours may be malignant cancers and they may reveal themselves as obvious lumps or swellings in the pelvis or abdomen. They can be visualised on an ultrasound scan or CAT scan of the pelvis and abdomen or by passing a telescope (laparoscope) through the abdominal wall.

Balding

Loss or thinning of the scalp hair is fairly common in women and usually causes a large amount of anxiety and stress. The medical term for loss of scalp hair is alopecia and, if it is associated with increased levels of male hormones, it is called 'androgenic alopecia'. Alopecia is frequently associated with increased levels of male hormones. The most common underlying cause for this disorder is polycystic ovarian syndrome and/or excess weight.

Androgenic alopecia may be of two types:

Male Pattern Androgenic Alopecia where the hair loss occurs in the areas of the crown, and temples and forehead, producing a receding hairline. Women with this type of alopecia may have inherited this tendency from their parents or grandparents.

Female Pattern Androgenic Alopecia where the hair loss is more diffuse or widespread. Hereditary factors are not as important in this type of hair loss. Female Pattern Androgenic Alopecia may occur around the time of the menopause, when the ovaries may increase their production of male hormones, while their output of the female hormones is slowing down.

The effect of male hormones upon scalp hair is opposite to their effect on facial and body hair. Whereas excessive male hormones increase facial and body hair, they reduce the growth of scalp hair. Excessive amounts or sensitivity to male hormones, may interfere with the scalp hair growth cycle and cause a progressive loss of strong, thick-coloured 'terminal' hair, which is replaced only by fine, soft 'vellus' hair, which resembles baby hair.

The Story of Heather

Heather, a 59-year old widow, had come to my surgery in a forlorn state. She had been consulting a dermatologist for several years to obtain treatment for hair loss from her scalp. When I examined her scalp, there was a definite loss of hair, as well as some circular areas on her scalp that had no hair at all. Heather had become anxious and had finally resorted to wearing a wig. She said that the steroid cortisone injections she was receiving into her scalp had been painful and ineffective.

Heather's hair loss had begun at the time of her natural menopause and she had also noticed an increase in unsightly facial hair at this time. Her blood sample revealed very low levels of oestrogen and elevated levels of free testosterone and a high Free Androgen Index (FAI). This is a common finding in the blood tests of post-menopausal women who are overweight and who are not receiving Hormone Replacement Therapy. I explained to Heather that she had 'Androgenic Alopecia' due to low levels of female hormones and excessive levels of male hormones (androgens).

Heather did not want to take oestrogen therapy so I started her on a course of Androcur (cyproterone acetate) tablets to reduce her level of male hormones. I also gave her nutritional supplements of cold pressed flaxseed oil, Selenium Complete and MSM Plus vitamin C powder and put her on a program of raw juicing; this would promote a glossy and healthy appearance to her skin and hair.

Nine months later, Heather's hair had improved dramatically and her male hormone levels were normal on her blood test results. It was unfortunate that two of the circular patches that had been injected with steroids did not respond and remained bald. I concluded that in general, it is best to avoid steroid injections into the scalp, unless all other measures had failed. Nevertheless, Heather was pleased with the result and was able to conceal her small bald circles by cleverly arranging her hair style. Heather was quite happy to continue the Androcur for many years, as it had stopped her facial hair and made her feel more feminine and attractive.

Acne

Male hormones stimulate the secretion of oily fluid from the skin's tiny glands, which are called sebaceous glands. In susceptible women, this may result in acne of various types and degrees, which begins at or soon after puberty and may persist well into the 20s and 30s and, in some cases, up to the menopause. Acne may be associated with raised levels of male hormones from the ovaries or adrenal glands, or may be due to an increased sensitivity of the skin's sebaceous glands to normal levels of male hormones. Women with polycystic ovaries often complain of moderate to severe acne along with their hirsutism.

Preventing the physical effects of too many hormones

Thankfully, it is now possible to prevent and reverse the masculine changes that result from excessive androgen production or sensitivity. In years gone by, acne and facial hair have caused women of all age groups considerable stress and embarrassment in their social and professional lives. Uncontrolled acne, in particular, may lead to permanent scarring and disfigurement if allowed to continue, but such women can now be promised near to perfect skin. I myself remember the extreme self-consciousness caused by my own adolescent acne and only wish that the doctor I had consulted way back then had known the valve of hormonal therapy in suppressing acne.

PROBLEMS	HORMONAL TREATMENT – suitable for all 3 problems in the left column of table	OTHER DRUGS AND MEASURES
1. Acne	1. Ethinyl oestradiol 20 to 50mcg daily with Androcur 2.5mg to 100mg for 2 or 3 weeks every month. 2. Aldactone 50 to 200mg daily or from day 5-26 of the menstrual cycle.	1. 'Roaccutane' tablets are extremely effective for cystic acne but because they can cause birth defects, they are only prescribed by skin specialists. 2. 'Retin A' cream or lotion – is also anti-ageing. 3. Long-term antibiotics (may cause candida) 4. Antibiotic lotion eg Neomedrol. 5. Selenium Complete tablets
2. Hirsutism (Excess Facial and/or Body Hair)	3. Oral contraceptive pill (OCP) by itself or with Androcur 2.5mg to 25mg daily or with Aldactone. 4. Androcur 12.5mg to 100mg daily by itself or with a natural oestrogen, in menopausal women, or women after hysterectomy.	Under the supervision of a beautician: Plucking – not recommended Waxing – not for very coarse thick hair Bleaching – for moustache Depilatory creams Shaving – does not increase hair regrowth Electrolysis – for small areas only Laser – can be very effective
3. Balding (Androgenic Alopecia)	5. Cortisone type drug, eg dexamethasone 0.25mg to 0.5mg at night.	Specific nutritional supplements may be very helpful such as: 1. MSM plus C powder 2. Flaxseed Oil – cold pressed 3. Raw juicing is vital 4. Kelp or culinary seaweeds 5. Calcium Complete (contains silica) Hair transplant therapy can work wonders Check function of thyroid gland

Footnote:
These are suggested schedules only and your doctor may vary them to suit your particular case. It is always worthwhile to consult a specialist dermatologist and a good beautician.

Overcoming acne and hirsutism

For women with moderate to severe acne or facial hair, it is usually necessary to use drugs with a hormonal action that will either reduce the body's production of male hormones and/or block the action of the male hormones upon the hair follicles and sebaceous glands in the skin. These drugs are extremely effective and, under strict medical supervision, are safe. They need to be given long term and you need to feel that the improvement in your appearance warrants the expense and slight risk in taking this long-term medication.

Because I am a naturopathic doctor, as well as a medical doctor, I am often asked if nutritional supplements can cure acne, facial hair or thinning of scalp hair. Unfortunately, they will not cure these problems and although they may help, particularly with thinning of scalp hair (see table on page 124), hormonal therapy is the most effective strategy.

Let us take a look at some of the hormonal drugs that reduce the production and action of the male hormones in our bodies.

Cyproterone

Cyproterone acetate is a remarkable drug that acts like an anti-male hormone as well as a progestogen

It is the most powerful anti-male hormone available providing an almost 100% cure of acne after three to nine months of use and reverses hirsutism in 80% of women after nine to twelve months of use. Approximately one in every two women with androgenic alopecia will obtain regrowth or thickening of the scalp hair after using cyproterone for nine to twelve months.

Cyproterone has been used overseas since 1974. Cyproterone can be used by itself and it is also a component of the oral contraceptive pill called 'Diane 35', which is commonly prescribed as a contraceptive in acne sufferers. Cyproterone is really a hormone with a dual action, being not only an anti-male hormone but also a progestogen, and so it exerts similar effects to progesterone and in particular can balance the effect of oestrogen upon the uterus.

Cyproterone can be given with the female hormone oestrogen on a cyclical basis, in much the same way as the oral contraceptive pill is taken. This can be tailor-made for you to suppress acne and/or facial hair and to provide contraception. In pre-menopausal women contraception is important, as women taking cyproterone must avoid pregnancy because its anti-male hormone properties may stop the sexual development in a male foetus. In post-menopausal women, or women who have had a hysterectomy, pregnancy is not a concern, and so cyproterone can be taken without regard to contraception.

Generally speaking, cyproterone is well tolerated by most women and, when it is given along with oestrogen, the side effects are similar to those of being on the oral contraceptive pill.

Most women are overjoyed to have clear feminine skin, which makes it easier to put up with any annoying side effects. Because cyproterone is a potent anti-male hormone, high doses of it may cause a reduction in sex drive, reduced concentration, fatigue and mild depression. Side effects can usually be avoided if the dosage of cyproterone is reduced. Once your skin is looking good, the dose can be reduced way down to around a ¼ of a tablet (12.5mg) daily, when side effects should disappear. In the long-term, the lowest possible dose that can keep your skin looking good should be used and your own doctor can guide you on this. Cyproterone is available as 50mg tablets on an authority prescription for women suffering with the effects of excessive male hormones and in such cases, is not expensive.

Aldactone

The chemical name for Aldactone is spironolactone and, like cyproterone, this is a drug with a dual action, being not only a diuretic but also an effective anti-male hormone. Aldactone is not as powerful in its anti-male hormone effects as cyproterone but may be sufficient for some women with facial hair, acne or balding. It is often preferable to use Aldactone rather than cyproterone in women with high blood pressure, fluid retention or severe depression or those who are troubled by a very low sex drive.

The amount of Aldactone needed to control acne and facial hair varies between different women. If breakthrough bleeding occurs or if contraception is required, Aldactone can be taken with the oral contraceptive pill. You must not become pregnant while taking Aldactone as, like cyproterone, Aldactone may cause feminisation of the developing male foetus.

Aldactone may cause minor side effects, such as breakthrough bleeding, slight breast enlargement, nausea, muscle cramps and an imbalance in potassium levels, but these may be avoided by reducing the dose.

Other Hormonal Treatments

In some women with mild acne and/or facial hair, a very good result can be obtained simply by taking the female hormone oestrogen. This will reduce the production of male hormones from the ovary and reduce production of oily secretions from the skin's sebaceous glands. In women with a uterus, it is also necessary to give progestogen to regulate menstrual bleeding and only progestogens without male (androgenic) properties should be used. Many of today's oral contraceptive pills contain androgenic progestogens such as norgestrel and norethisterone and these should be avoided, as they may worsen acne and facial hair. The best types of Oral Contraceptive Pills (OCP) for women with acne and/or facial hair are those which contain progestogens that have an anti-male hormone or feminine effect. Examples of these brands are Diane, Brenda, Juliet, Femoden, Trioden, Minulet, Marvelon and Yasmin; these will greatly improve acne and skin texture.

Menopausal and post menopausal women with facial hair often find that the natural oestrogen in their **hormone replacement therapy** greatly reduces this problem, especially if a small dose of Androcur or Aldactone is added.

Excessive male hormone production from the adrenal glands can be suppressed by taking a very small dose of a **cortisone-type preparation**, such as dexamethasone once a night upon retiring. One should use only the smallest possible dose of cortisone-type drugs as an impaired response to stress may occur.

The Story of Julia

Timely hormonal therapy may help to avoid unnecessary surgery, as was the case for Julia, a 32-year old woman, who came to see me complaining of symptoms typical of **polycystic ovarian disorder**. Since the birth of her son eight years ago, she had developed PMT, facial hair and acne. Julia had bouts of sharp pelvic pains and an ultrasound scan of her pelvis revealed enlarged ovaries with many small cysts around their periphery. She had consulted a surgeon, who told her that the only option was to remove her left ovary and take a wedge of tissue out of her right ovary. Julia was alarmed at this prospect because she did not want to lose an ovary this early in life. She consulted another doctor, who prescribed a low-dose oral contraceptive pill but unfortunately, it contained an androgenic progestogen and did not help her facial hair and acne. We discussed the possibility of suppressing her androgen producing ovarian cysts with oestrogen and Androcur and she was delighted to learn that Androcur would cure her acne and facial hair. I prescribed Estigyn .05mg and Androcur 50mg for two weeks every month and advised her to avoid surgery as her ovarian cysts were typical of polycystic ovaries and not a tumour or cancer. After six months of Estigyn and Androcur, Julia's ovaries had returned to their normal size, their cysts had become much smaller and her skin was clear and much more feminine in appearance. Julia also found the treatment very convenient as it provided her with reliable contraception.

The Story of Barbara

Excessive secretion of male hormones associated with **polycystic ovaries** is quite common and can be responsible for much suffering and confusion, which was exactly the case for 34-year old Barbara, who had been trying to become pregnant for more than two years. Barbara's menstrual cycle had always been infrequent and irregular and, every three or four months, she would have a menstrual flow that was heralded by PMT, large blind pimples and depression. Since the age of 18, she had developed facial hair and gradually gained excessive weight. Her mother said it was all the fault of her diet and that if she gave up fats and sugars, her pimples would clear. Barbara's mother's surprise was only surpassed by Barbara's relief when I explained that her problems were due to excessive levels of male hormones.

I referred Barbara to an infertility specialist so that she could receive fertility drugs to stimulate regular ovulation in her polycystic ovaries. Barbara became pregnant with the fertility drugs and nine months after the birth of her daughter came to see me, as her polycystic ovaries were once again over-producing male hormones. Subsequently, Barbara's facial hair and acne were very well controlled with Diane and extra Androcur and a weight-loss programme.

The Story of Susan

Susan, an actress, comedienne and singer was understandably very concerned with keeping her skin at its best. In her early 30s her hormonal balance changed after having had three children and she developed **'mature aged acne'.**

She became quite obsessed when, every month before her period, several blind pimples would appear on her chin and forehead and her husband and children complained to me that she sounded like a broken record. In her eyes, the pimples were like volcanos and she resorted to wearing bandaids on her face to conceal them. Her family and friends could hardly see these few pimples and told her that she was being overly anxious.

I referred Susan to a hormone specialist (endocrinologist), who began her on Aldactone tablets. These helped her acne but caused annoying breakthrough bleeding. Her specialist then tried Androcur and oestrogen tablets, but Susan was not able to tolerate oestrogen in oral (tablet) form as it caused nausea.

Her endocrinologist was by this time understanding that actresses are highly strung and sensitive creatures and racked his brains for an alternative to facial bandaids.

He suggested to Susan that she try oestrogen in injection form and so she began a course of monthly Primogyn Depot injections, each one being given at the end of her menstrual bleeding. Much to the relief of the doctor and Susan's family, this stopped the mild acne and she stopped wearing bandaids on her beautiful face.

It may seem minor to you but it is another example of how only a minor imbalance in the ratio of female to male hormones can cause small or large physical changes that, in an individual, can have ruinous effects.

For women, who over-produce male hormones, therapy with oestrogen and anti-male hormones can be dramatically effective. These treatments are slow acting with nine to twelve months of therapy being needed for a total relief of symptoms. However, it is not a cure and symptoms such as acne, hirsutism and balding usually return several months after hormonal therapy is stopped. For permanent control, it is usually necessary to continue treatment on a long-term basis with interruption if pregnancy is desired.

These hormonal treatments should not be started before the sexual development and longitudinal growth spurt of adolescence is completed, otherwise, a reduction in the attainment of height may occur. Furthermore, therapy needs to be guided under strict medical supervision and regular blood tests.

Hormonal Imbalances and weight gain

There is no doubt that hormonal imbalances can cause a weight problem. Years ago doctors, family members and friends would often advise women who battled with a weight problem that it was due to "hormonal problems" or their "glands". In those days there was very little understanding about the ways that hormones affected the body. No real help was available and the patient just accepted that this was the way she had to remain.

Today things have improved greatly and we now know that specific hormones such as insulin, thyroid hormones, androgens and oestrogens can affect metabolism, and also the areas where excessive fat will be deposited. We are able to measure accurately the blood levels of all the body's hormones, and can pin point the significant hormonal imbalances that will trigger weight gain.

Your body type or body shape is affected by your hormones. For example oestrogen causes fat to be deposited in the lower part of the body in the hips, buttocks and thighs. Fat in the lower part of the body also produces a type of oestrogen called oestrone, which can lead to cellulite in this area. This type of cellulite can be reduced with a high dose brindleberry formula containing 5500mg of brindleberry per tablet. The addition of kelp, chromium, zinc, B6, and tyrosine make the brindleberry more effective in burning fat. It is necessary to take 1 tablet, 3 times daily, just before meals. For more information call the Health Advisory Service on 02 4655 8855

Androgens cause fat to be deposited in the upper part of the body (above the hips) so that weight gain occurs in the trunk and abdomen. Fat in the upper part of the body produces androgens and if these androgens are very high, weight loss becomes much harder.

If you would like to do an interactive questionnaire to determine which of the four body types you belong to – visit www.weightcontroldoctor.com and get your answer – you will find it fascinating! This web site explains the four different body types and their unique hormonal and metabolic differences, which explains where you put on weight most easily. For a comprehensive calorie controlled diet to suit your body type see my book titled "The Body Shaping Diet" which enables you to lose weight from where you really need to and want to.

Thyroid Gland Dysfunction

Dysfunction of the thyroid gland can have a profound effect on the metabolism. An overactive thyroid gland produces excess amounts of thyroid hormone, which results in weight loss, even though there is a voracious appetite. Conversely, an under active thyroid gland does not produce adequate amounts of thyroid hormone and the metabolism slows down. *The symptoms of thyroid gland underactivity are*

Weight gain with a very slow metabolism

Fluid retention & puffiness

Bloating & constipation

Low body temperature

Depression and mental slowness

Muscle weakness & wasting

Hair loss and Dryness of the skin

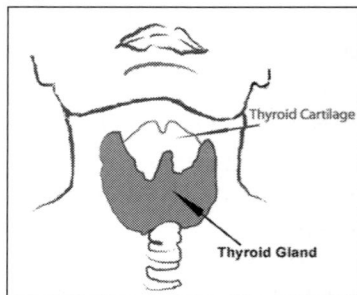

Thyroid Cartilage

Thyroid Gland

The condition of thyroid gland underactivity is called Hypothyroidism, while the condition of an overactive thyroid gland is called Hyperthyroidism.

Hypothyroidism is very common in middle aged persons, especially perimenopausal women. It is associated with fatigue and muscle weakness, so there is not much inclination to exercise, which leads to more weight gain.

The function of the thyroid gland can be easily checked with a simple blood test, which measures the level of the thyroid hormones. The thyroid gland produces the hormone called thyroxine, which is also known as T4. Thyroxine (T4) must be converted in the body into the more active form of thyroid hormone, which is known as triiodothyronine or T3. The active form of thyroid hormone (T3) directly stimulates the energy factories inside the cells to burn food calories at a faster rate. This is why those with an over-active thyroid gland lose weight, even though they are eating much more than normal.

The blood tests for thyroid gland function must measure at least the following three hormones

HORMONE	NORMAL RANGE
Thyroid Stimulating Hormone (TSH)	(0.5 to 5.0) mIU/L
Free T 4	(9.0 to 24.0) pmol/L
Free T 3	(2.2 to 5.4) pmol/L

If the T 4 and/or T 3 levels are found to be below the normal ranges, and the TSH is found to be above the normal range, we can say that the thyroid gland is under active.

If the thyroid gland is only slightly under active, we are often able to stimulate it back to normal function by the following

- Improving the diet and lifestyle
- Taking supplemental magnesium tablets
- Taking supplemental selenium 100 to 200mcg daily (Ref 31,32)
- Taking supplemental flaxseed oil and evening primrose oil

If however the thyroid function remains abnormally low after 3 months of nutritional supplementation, it will be necessary to take thyroid hormone replacement. This is usually given in the form of tablets containing thyroxine hormone. Many people worry that taking thyroxine tablets is the same as taking artificial drugs, however this is not correct, as thyroxine tablets are merely replacing a natural hormone that the thyroid gland can no longer produce by itself. If the dosage is carefully controlled, there are generally no side effects.

In most people the thyroxine tablets work very well and increase the metabolic rate back to normal, so that weight loss begins and energy levels are restored.

In some people the thyroxine tablets have a good initial response, but become increasingly ineffective over time. This condition is called "thyroid resistance", and means that the body cells have become resistant to the effect of the hormone thyroxine (T4).

Thyroid Resistance

The term "thyroid resistance" describes the condition of a patient who is taking thyroid medication and yet despite this, is still experiencing the symptoms of an under-active thyroid gland. Obviously the patient is not responding adequately to the thyroid medication, or in other words is resistant to the thyroid medication. The condition of thyroid resistance is not uncommon and is responsible for a lot of chronic physical symptoms and psychological frustration. Unfortunately many sufferers find it difficult to get the help they need to overcome thyroid resistance. I am aware of this because I see plenty of patients with this problem and they also write or email our Health Advisory Service about it.

What causes thyroid resistance?

1. Lack of conversion

The patient is not able to convert the thyroid medication into its more active form. Most patients with an under-active thyroid gland are given thyroid hormone in the form of thyroxine or T 4. This must be converted into a more active form of thyroid hormone known as triiodothyronine or T 3. Triiodothyronine is around 10 times more active than T 4, and is much more effective than T 4 in speeding up the metabolism thus enhancing energy levels and weight loss.

Thyroid resistance is more common in patients who have had their whole thyroid gland surgically removed, or who have had radioactive iodine therapy or radiation therapy to the area of the neck where the thyroid gland is situated.

The reduced ability to convert T 4 into the more potent T 3 may be due to deficiencies of minerals such as selenium, zinc, magnesium or iodine, and selenium is the most common mineral to be found deficient in these patients. In some patients we cannot find a cause for the reduced ability of the body to convert the T 4 into T 3.

2. Poor cell response

In some patients there is a poor response of the body's cells to the thyroid hormone despite the use of increasing doses of thyroxine (T 4) tablets. This can be due to a lack of receptors for the thyroid hormones on the cell membranes. For some reason the cells do not produce adequate numbers of receptors to attract and attach the thyroid hormone to. The receptors may also be of poor quality if the cell membranes are unhealthy. The cell membranes and/or their receptors could be damaged from such things as auto-antibodies, viruses, radiation or deficiencies of vital nutrients. Deficiencies of essential fatty acids and antioxidant vitamins and minerals can lead to unhealthy cell membranes. Diabetics or those with Syndrome X have elevated blood sugar levels, which can impair the function and structure of their cell membranes, and thus they become prone to hormonal resistance.

Blood tests for thyroid resistance

If thyroid resistance is suspected it is important to have a blood test that will check the levels of ALL the thyroid hormones – namely TSH, free T 4 and free T 3.

If your body is not efficiently converting the T 4 into T 3, your doctor will find that the level of free T 3 in your blood test is abnormally low. In such cases your T 4 levels will be normal or even high, and your TSH levels may be normal or elevated. The important thing to find in cases of poor conversion is a low level of free T 3 – that clinches the diagnosis!

If your TSH level is elevated, and the levels of free T 4 are lower than normal, you are not receiving an adequate dosage of T 4 (thyroxine) tablets and your doctor needs to increase the dose of your thyroxine tablets.

If all your blood levels of thyroid hormones (free T 4, free T 3, and TSH) are normal, you probably have the type of thyroid resistance that is due to poor cell response to the thyroid hormones.

Symptoms of thyroid resistance

These are similar to the symptoms of under-activity of the thyroid gland also known as hypothyroidism. They may include –
- Weight excess & inability to lose weight
- Dry skin and hair
- Hair loss from the scalp
- Weakness of the muscles
- Fatigue
- Constipation

- Mental slowness and depression
- Shortness of breath
- Poor exercise tolerance

Because the thyroid resistant patient appears to be "thyroid under-active", she/he is often given excess doses of thyroxine (T 4), however this will not work very well, as the patient is unable to respond to the T 4. The very high doses of T 4 may cause the patient to become toxic, which causes agitation, racing heart beat, palpitations, muscle weakness, poor sleep and fatigue. In such cases the dose of T 4 needs to be reduced, and some T 3 tablets plus nutritional supplements, need to be given.

Treatment of thyroid resistance

In patients who are poor converters of T 4 into T 3 we can first try a course of nutritional supplements to increase the conversion.

I suggest the following

- Selenium 100 to 200 mcg daily
  (use the organic form of selenomethionine)
- Magnesium Complete – 2 to 4 tablets daily
- Kelp or other seaweeds (arame, wakame, dulse, kombu, nori) can
  be included in the diet – see your health food store. These culinary
  seaweeds are very high in trace minerals and can be used in stir-fries,
  salads, soups, stews etc.

If after several months of nutritional supplementation, the blood levels of free T 3 are still abnormally low, we need to add another type of thyroid hormone tablet to the thyroxine tablets. This is called Tertroxin and contains pure T 3 (known as triiodothyronine). This usually works very well and typical doses are 10mcg (1/2 tablet), 2 to 3 times daily. Tertroxin must be given more often than thyroxine because the body uses it up much more quickly. You will still need to continue your thyroxine (T 4) tablets, although your doctor will probably eventually need to reduce the dosage of thyroxine, often considerably, once the effect of the tertroxin kicks in. In patients who really need tertroxin the benefits quickly become obvious and the patient notices a large, and sometimes dramatic improvement in their well being.

If the addition of Tertroxin to the Thyroxine tablets does not produce a relief of the symptoms, then it is worthwhile to consult a doctor who can prescribe "natural thyroid extract" which is made from animal thyroid glands; this is available in Australia from some compounding pharmacists. In the USA this natural thyroid extract is called armour thyroid – see www.armour.com

You will still need a doctor's script for natural thyroid extract because like all types of thyroid hormones, its dose needs to be carefully controlled to achieve the correct levels in the blood.

In patients with symptoms of thyroid resistance, who have normal blood levels of all the thyroid hormones, we need to work on improving the cell membranes and their receptors, so that we can improve the cell's response to thyroid hormones.

If you are overweight or have high blood sugar levels and Syndrome X, it is important to lose weight and I recommend that you follow the eating plan in chapter 23 of my book titled *"Can't Lose Weight? – you could have Syndrome X"*

> **I also recommend supplements to improve the health of your cell membranes and these include –**
> - Essential fatty acids from oily fish, salmon oil, avocadoes, cold pressed flaxseed oil and raw nuts and seeds
> - The antioxidants selenium, zinc, vitamin E and vitamin C. Raw juices will provide high doses of phyto-nutrient antioxidants to improve your cell membranes.

To illustrate just how destructive undiagnosed thyroid resistance can be in someone's life, I would like to share with you a case history of a patient who had severe thyroid resistance.

Mary's Story

Mary was 46 years of age and had been unwell since she had undergone a total surgical removal of her thyroid gland 12 years ago. She was taking a huge dose of thyroxine (T 4) tablets of 400mcg daily and found that it did not relieve her symptoms.

Mary complained of –

Inability to lose weight – she was 5 foot 5 inches in height and weighed 110 kilograms despite being a life long member of weight watchers, and she did not believe that she ate excess amounts of food

Depression because of her appearance

Facial hair which was related to the excess amount of male hormones produced by the large amounts of fat she had accumulated in the upper parts of her body and her abdomen

Severe chronic fatigue although the large amounts of thyroxine were making her feel "hyped-up"

Poor libido

Mary had complained of these symptoms repetitively over many years to several doctors who had done blood tests to check her thyroid levels. The doctors had responded by giving her more and more thyroxine until she became toxic, and then they had to reduce the dose again, so she felt as though she was on a see-saw of highs and lows. Mary felt that she had never been on the correct dose for any length of time and felt helpless. She hated her appearance and desperately wanted to lose weight, but the weight would not budge. Mary also noticed that her eyes were bulging and swollen, which was due to the fact that she had had an auto-immune disease of her thyroid gland called Grave's disease. This had been the original reason that she had to have her thyroid gland removed.

Mary tried to be happy; she reminded herself that she had a wonderful husband, three lovely sons, and a good job and lived in a beautiful part of Australia. She gave herself positive affirmations which kept her going for a while, but then she would catch her reflection in a shop window and wonder who the fat lady with her outfit on was. Her friends did not always recognize her, or would ask rude questions like "Oh my God, what have you done to yourself". Yes its true people can be so ignorant and rude sometimes!

Mary became so obsessed with her weight that she went on a liquid diet for 4 months and lost 18 kilograms. This caused her to become so weak that she could not turn on the kitchen tap. Once she started eating normally again she put all the weight back on and started talking to her husband about a stomach stapling operation. However they both worked out that she did not eat enough to justify the risk and expense of this operation.

Mary was correct – she did not need a stomach stapling operation, as this would not have corrected her hormonal imbalance.

What Mary needed was treatment of her thyroid resistance with the addition of tertroxin (T 3) tablets to her thyroxine (T 4) tablets. This would have enabled her doctor to reduce the dose of her thyroxine tablets to reasonable levels to prevent her from becoming toxic. The tertroxin tablets would have provided the T 3 that her body was unable to produce from the T 4 tablets. This would have relieved her symptoms and enabled her to lose weight easily. She could have also achieved a good result by using natural thyroid extract tablets. I would have encouraged Mary to follow my Syndrome X eating plan to correct her metabolism and I would have prescribed a supplement containing selenium and zinc as well as some culinary seaweeds. Such a simple and safe solution to a long and painful illness is possible only if we understand the importance of fine-tuning our hormones. Thankfully Mary did not give up, and I was able to tell her face to face exactly what she needed to do, as she met me one day during one of my seminars in rural Australia.

The Adrenal Gland

The adrenal gland manufactures hormones that are secreted into the blood stream. The adrenal gland is divided into two parts - the inner part (know as the medulla) and the outer part (known as the cortex) - see page 138. These two parts are really like two separate organs because they are made of different types of tissue, which have different functions. The adrenal medulla manufactures the hormone called adrenaline when we are put under stress.

The outer layer of the adrenal gland, or cortex, manufactures about 30 different steroid hormones, but only a few are secreted in large amounts. One of these hormones is called Aldosterone and regulates the blood pressure and balance of salt and water in the body. The adrenal cortex also manufactures cortisol, which is used to regulate the metabolism of fats, carbohydrates, and proteins.

Overactive adrenal glands can make us hairy and masculine in appearance if they over produce male hormones. Adrenal gland dysfunction can have even more devastating effects upon the appearance if they over-produce the hormone cortisol. Excessive adrenal gland production of cortisol results in 'Cushing's Syndrome' causing a rare but horrible collection of physical changes. As with most hormonal disorders, the physical changes appear gradually and may be mistakenly attributed to diet, lifestyle or age.

In Cushing's Syndrome, changes to the physique can make it resemble an 'orange on toothpicks' with a fat trunk, a 'buffalo hump' at the back of the neck, a round moon-shaped face and skinny muscle-wasted limbs! The skin may also be affected and becomes thin with purple stretch marks and increased bruising and facial hair.

The most common cause of Cushing's Syndrome is the long-term administration of cortisone tablets to treat conditions, such as arthritis or asthma, and so doctors always try to give their patients the smallest possible dose of these life-saving drugs. Cushing's Syndrome may also occur because of a tumour of the pituitary or adrenal gland.

The amount of cortisol produced by your adrenal glands is easily checked with blood and urine tests. If a tumour of the pituitary or adrenal gland is discovered, surgical treatment may be required.

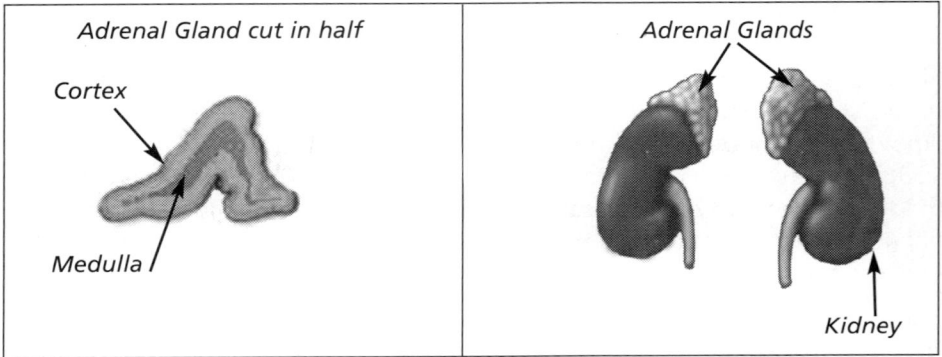

Adrenal Gland cut in half

Cortex

Medulla

Adrenal Glands

Kidney

The Pituitary Gland

The pituitary gland may cause major changes in appearance if it over-produces growth hormone in adult life after normal growth has ceased. This is not a common occurrence, which is fortunate as the effects of excessive growth hormone on the skull, feet and hands may enlarge them considerably requiring a change in the size of hats, gloves and shoes. The length of the bones will not increase but the soft tissues of the body and cartilage of the joints will enlarge, causing an increase in the size of the jaw and nose so that the face will eventually assume a coarse, heavy-featured look with a protruding jaw line.

The physical condition caused by excessive growth hormone is called Acromegaly. Because these changes occur slowly, once again, they may be mistakenly put down to overeating or getting older, especially as Acromegaly is uncommon.

The cause of this condition is usually a tumour of the pituitary gland, which could be cured by surgery.

Cushing's Syndrome and Acromegaly are awful diseases but, luckily, they are the rare and extreme cases – the most terrible results of how hormones can affect your appearance.

CHAPTER 11

Hormones and your sex life

Many women have consulted me over the years, revealing their sexual frustrations and problems and it has been a shock to see how difficult it can be to find practical solutions to these problems.

Ideally, as a woman ages, she becomes more relaxed as a sexual being, realising that the most important thing about sex is that ideally it can be fun and stress-relieving. She is also more knowledgeable about her own individual needs and what it takes to give her sexual satisfaction. Maturity enables her to be more easily assertive and effective in asking to have her needs fulfilled. Many women have told me that their sexual desire increases as they age and for some of them, there is more sexual interest, pleasure and capacity for orgasm. Women are living longer and may out live their partners or find new relationships which need nurturing.

As a doctor, I have found that many women have huge fluctuations in libido (sex drive) and enjoyment of sex, especially as they are approaching the menopause.

When the levels of the sex hormones of both male and female variety are low, the sex drive will suffer. This may occur for six to twelve months after childbirth and also gradually after the age of 45 to 50 years as the menopause approaches. If the levels of the sex hormones are low, there may also be a change in the personality and a woman may become disinterested and unresponsive and shun the advances of the man she has previously loved and desired.

It is sad when these problems in older women disrupt an otherwise good relationship or marriage. This is unnecessary because early help could salvage both the woman's sexuality and the man's ego. Then, divorce rates and the number of lonely middle aged people would definitely decrease.

It is interesting for me as a doctor to find that poor libido or sex drive is a common problem in women. No one ever complains about have too much libido and indeed it seems for some, the more the better!

The greatest destroyers of libido include:

1. Insufficient production of the male and female sex hormones. This can be aggravated by an unhealthy lifestyle and diet and laboratory

testing shows that men and women, who drink and/or smoke excessively, have lower levels of sex hormones in their blood. Women, who smoke heavily, are more prone to an early menopause, which will further reduce their libido.

2. In men, the fear of poor performance or premature ejaculation causes stress and reduces libido. Thankfully, women are far less prone to this type of stress however any type of chronic stress or depression can greatly reduce the sex drive.

3. Menopausal women are susceptible to vaginal shrinkage and dryness and so may experience pain during sexual intercourse. Furthermore, if shrinkage of the vulva and clitoris occurs, normal lubrication and orgasmic capacity becomes very difficult. Understandably, many menopausal and post menopausal women in this situation avoid sexual contact.

4. Various prescription medications may reduce libido. Take the example of Peter, a 44-year old, aggressive business executive. Despite normal ups and downs in their sixteen years of marriage, he and his wife had never had sexual problems until Peter accepted drug treatment for ulcer pains. Despite his strong desires, he is discouraged to find that his erections no longer last. Or take the case of Christine, who has started anti-depressant medication for her chronic depression. Although her moods and libido have returned to normal, she is frustrated by her inability to achieve orgasm. It is now increasingly recognised that situations such as those of Peter and Christine are common. A wide range of drugs may affect sexual function causing loss of libido, arousal difficulty, orgasmic dysfunction or reproductive impairment. The most common drugs to cause these problems are appetite suppressants, some muscle relaxants, some drugs for epilepsy, some drugs to prevent headaches, some drugs to treat high blood pressure, some sedatives and anti-depressants, some anti-ulcer drugs and some hormones, particularly anti-male hormones. Make sure you check with your doctor before you're given a new medication, as you may be in for a surprise when your sexual ability and desire become reduced through the medication. There is often a suitable alternative drug, which will not do this, as new derivatives of older drugs, which have a lesser incidence of side effects, are becoming available every day.

5. Boredom and routine may creep into a long-term relationship, especially if the male partner is unaware of the needs and changes in the sexuality of a woman as she ages. He may not realise that he will need to be gentler and take more time to stimulate his partner before entry.

What to do for a poor libido

If you find yourself in the quandary of poor libido and loss of sexual enjoyment and performance, which is disrupting a valuable relationship, see your doctor for a thorough medical checkup to see if there is any physical disorder or disease that could be causing this situation. Such disorders are thyroid imbalance, high blood pressure, diabetes, hardening of the arteries, lower back problems or diseases of the nervous system, such as multiple sclerosis. If, after a thorough physical examination, your doctor cannot find any obvious physical causes to explain your problem, the next step is to have the level of the sex hormones measured in your blood. If these levels are low or borderline (at the lower limit of the normal range), you should benefit greatly from specific Hormone Replacement Therapy.

It may require a little time, patience and experimentation with different types of hormones to find the right combination to turn you on. Some combinations and types of synthetic hormones will frankly turn you off and for this reason, women, who have been taking the synthetic hormones found in the oral contraceptive pill for some time, often experience a reduction in libido. Similarly, some menopausal and pre-menopausal women find that conventional HRT with oestrogen and synthetic progesterone does not recapture their former enjoyment of sex.

General measures to help a poor libido

You and your doctor have several alternatives to play with to encourage the libido and I will qualify these with my own clinical results. The use of conventional tablet forms of HRT containing natural oestrogens and synthetic progesterone will restore the capacity for a normal sex life in the majority of women suffering with a sex hormone deficiency during menopause. In addition, for those women with a dry over-sensitive or fragile vagina that fails to lubricate adequately, the use of oestrogen creams applied to the vagina and vaginal lips (vulva) can be extremely beneficial. Many women with these problems turn to bland creams or jellies, such as 'KY jelly', but these only have a temporary lubricating action.

Conversely, hormonal creams restore and rejuvenate the mucosal lining of the vagina and vulva and improve the circulation of blood to the clitoral area, thus restoring the capacity for natural lubrication and orgasm. (Diagram 20 on page 143). Some of my patients have told me that hormonal creams act like an aphrodisiac and make them feel very sexy.

Some menopausal women have shrinkage of the vagina, vulva and clitoris and painful scar tissue forming in the roof of the vagina, which can make it impossible for the penis to penetrate without pain. These problems can be overcome by regularly massaging the vulva with a hormonal cream and gently stretching apart the vaginal walls with your fingers. This can be done gradually more and more each day, and there is no need to stretch excessively and cause pain. In some women, particularly those who have undergone a premature menopause, shrinkage of the vulva and clitoris can be extreme and, in these cases, a hormone cream can be massaged gently into the vulva and clitoris twice daily. A compounding pharmacist can make up the hormone cream especially for you according to your doctor's prescription.

A typical hormone cream would contain the following combination and amounts of hormones

- Natural oestrogen (oestradiol) 1 to 2mg
- Natural progesterone 40mg
- Natural testosterone 2mg

All in one cream! Now that's practical and cost saving.

Vaginal discomfort and pain

Most cases of vaginal dryness and discomfort are due to a lack of oestrogen, which can occur during the menopause and also after childbirth. This is usually totally relieved with the use of hormonal creams applied to the vulva and vaginal areas. In some women, the vulva becomes very dry, itchy and painful and the lips of the vagina become pale, shrunken and chronically inflamed. This is not a normal condition and is caused by immune dysfunction. This condition is called lichen sclerosis of the vulva and is not healthy, as it can be pre-malignant. If you suspect that you have this condition I recommend that you see a specialist gynaecologist as a biopsy (small sample) of the affected tissue must be taken and checked under a microscope. In lichen sclerosis of the vulva and/or vagina, nutritional supplements can reduce the discomfort and heal the inflammation. Indeed if the condition is picked up early enough it is not difficult to cure it, although regular 12 monthly follow up from your doctor is still advised.

The appropriate supplements to take are-

Cold pressed flaxseed oil – 3 tsp daily
Organic selenium 100mcg daily
Zinc 20mg daily (as zinc amino acid chelate)
Vitamin E 200 IU and Vitamin C 500-1000mg daily

These are available combined together in one tablet

For more information call the Women's Health Advisory Service on 0246 55 8855

- Raw vegetable juices are also extremely helpful – you can combine carrot, apple, cabbage, beetroot and capsicum and orange for an anti-oxidant packed healing juice

Lichen sclerosis of the vulva and/or vagina will also require the use of a cream containing natural hormones, especially in older women, or women who are deficient in sex hormones. Suitable creams can be made up by a compounding pharmacist to contain mixtures of natural oestrogen, progesterone and testosterone. These creams are applied to the affected area every day after washing.

If recurrent infections of the vagina, vulva or bladder complicate the problem, bathing the area in a very weak dilution of tea tree oil douche gel, instead of soap is useful. If infection with candida is present, make sure that you avoid bread, yeast, sugar and foods high in refined carbohydrates.

To eradicate candida and other infections, you may add small amounts of raw garlic and horseradish to red apple and carrot and pass them all through the juicer. If you hate garlic, add red onion instead. Make sure that you add plenty of carrot and apple to temper the flavour.

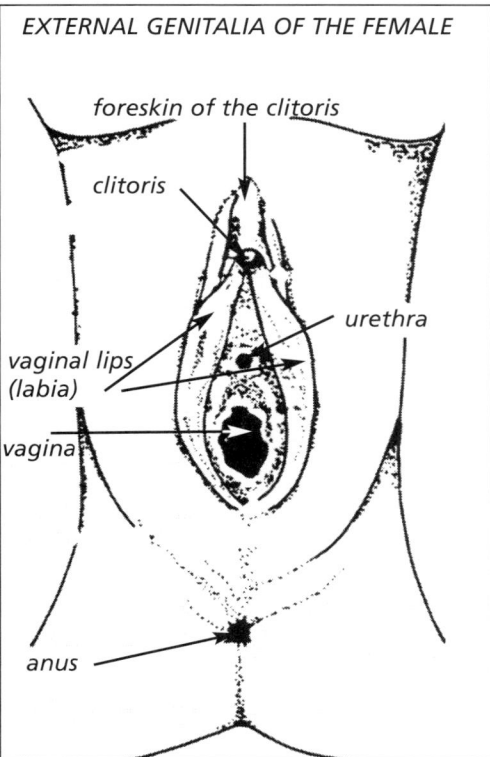

EXTERNAL GENITALIA OF THE FEMALE

foreskin of the clitoris

clitoris

urethra

vaginal lips (labia)

vagina

anus

Hormone therapy to improve the sex life

For various reasons some women, especially during menopause, experience a total loss of libido, even to the point where they become "frigid" or cannot tolerate any sexual advances or even affection from their partner. In such cases counselling from a sex therapist is often helpful.

Conventional hormone replacement therapy using oestrogen

and progesterone tablets may not be able to overcome the problem satisfactorily. As a temporary solution these women may find that injections of natural oestrogen can produce a return of a healthy libido and increased mental and physical wellbeing. These injections can be very helpful for women experiencing a total loss of libido associated with severe anxiety and depression and are also effective in overcoming loss of libido and depression after a hysterectomy.

These injections are oily and need to be given deeply into the muscles of the buttock, where they provide a storage or depot of hormone that will be slowly released into the blood for a four to five week period. Thus, these injections will need to be repeated approximately every five to six weeks.

An oestrogen injection is available under the brand name of Primogyn Depot. These injections are a potent form of oestrogen, even though it is natural oestrogen, and thus their use cannot be recommended for more than several months at a time. Otherwise excessive blood levels of oestrogen may result with an attendant increased risk of hormone dependent cancers.

A healthy sex drive or libido in women is equally dependent upon sufficient amounts of female and male hormones. These days, male hormones are being used more and more to complement the replacement of the female hormones, oestrogen and progesterone in menopausal and post menopausal women. Natural male hormones may be administered in the form of a testosterone cream and may be just what's needed to lift a sexual low or crisis. The physiological effects of male hormones are to increase the size and sensitivity of the clitoris, which may have been very tiny, about the size of a match head. After the use of a testosterone cream on the vulva and clitoris for several weeks, there will be an increased responsiveness to sexual stimulation, either partner or self-induced. Male hormones may increase the intensity and frequency of orgasms or enable a woman to have an orgasm for the first time in her life! The result can be astonishing and women, who have always found sex a bore or a chore, may change after two to six weeks, and thereafter progression often occurs without further hormone therapy. Sexual pleasure and arousal may set off hormonal changes that are self-perpetuating. Patients on hormone therapy may start to have sexy dreams and dress in a more provocative way.

Many women worry that male hormones will turn them into hairy amazons, and are too frightened to try them! If male hormones are used in excessive dosage, they can cause facial hair, slight weight gain, greasy pimply skin, and sometimes deepening of the voice. Older women may notice a desirable increase in pubic hair. Thankfully, the desired effects of male hormones usually occur before unwanted side effects appear. If male hormones are taken in small doses in the form of creams, these possible side effects should be minimal, and are usually non-existent, and if they do occur they will only be temporary. It is important to avoid pregnancy during hormone treatment for sexual problems and for four weeks after finishing treatment.

I personally believe that the use of natural male hormones in the form of creams is extremely useful in the situation where a woman's libido and sexuality is at such a low ebb that she can no longer cope or her marriage is about the collapse. A cream containing a combination of natural oestrogen, progesterone and testosterone can be dramatically effective in increasing sexual, mental and emotional wellbeing and pull a woman out of an otherwise endless pit.

Needless to say, it is essential that women undergo these hormonal treatments only under the careful supervision of a doctor, who is interested and experienced in women's health. Before any type of Hormone Replacement Therapy is commenced, whether it is in the form of tablets, creams, implants or injections, a thorough general check up and a screening for breast and gynaecological cancer must be painstakingly performed and

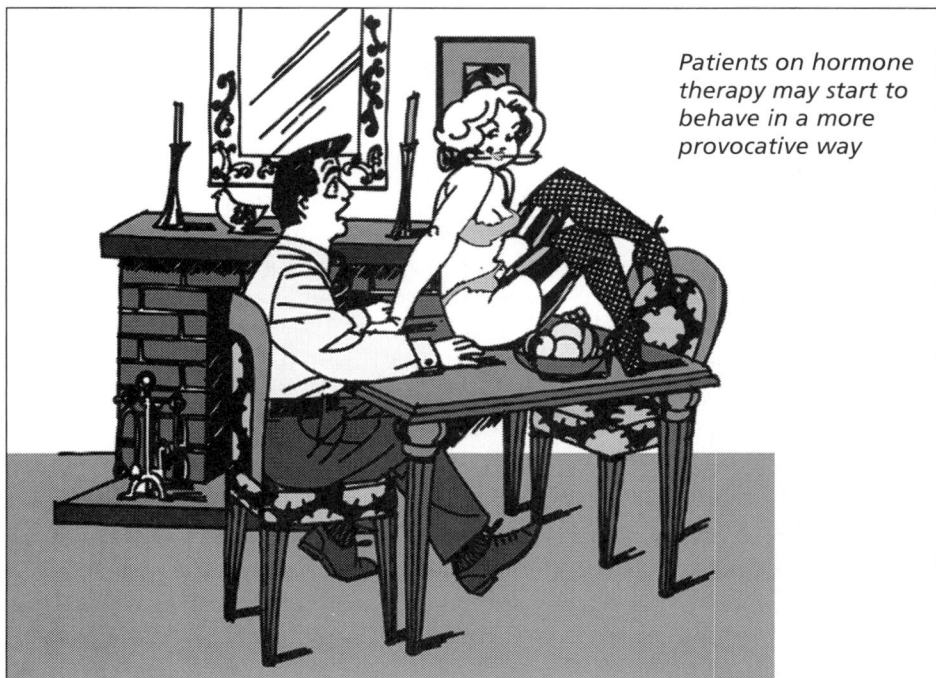

Patients on hormone therapy may start to behave in a more provocative way

repeated every twelve months. This is because an early silent cancer of the breast or uterus could be stimulated by hormone replacement therapy.

The Male Menopause – fact or fiction?

This section is designed for you and your partner if he has a midlife crisis.

The word 'menopause' literally means the cessation of menstrual bleeding. In females, it signifies that the biological clock has stopped and infertility sets in accompanied by dramatic hormonal changes. So, the word, 'menopause' cannot apply to men. Yet, even though they seem to be on easy street compared to women, it is indeed a fact that men also are vulnerable to emotional, mental and physical changes at about 50 years of age and beyond when Hormone Replacement Therapy (HRT) may be of help to men as well as women.

The first semblance of Hormone Replacement Therapy (HRT) was used in a man in 1889, when a famous neurophysiologist professor Charles-Edouard Brown-Sequard, gave himself an extract of animal testicles. In his own words, this produced 'a return of vigour, youthful appetites and desires' due to the male hormone testosterone contained in the animal testicles.

Hormonal changes in men

Testosterone production from the testicles is at its peak during the 20s and 30s and thereafter, a slow decline occurs, which becomes more apparent after the age of 50. Despite this, there is a large variation between individual males so that some men at 50 may produce such low levels of testosterone that they no longer feel any inclination to have a sex life, whereas others at 80 have high testosterone levels and are still sexually vigorous. As you are reading this, you are probably wondering how you (if you are a male) or your partner can be one of the lucky ones and nurture those testicles all the way along throughout life. The ability to produce testosterone is partly genetic so that in many cases, it's 'like father, like son'. We also know that lifestyle plays a role and men, who are overweight, smoke and/or drink alcohol excessively, will have lower levels of testosterone in their blood.

As a man ages, not only does the production of testosterone diminish, but so does the ability of his tissues and cells to respond to testosterone. It is a simple matter for a man to see if his testosterone production is down by asking for a blood test.

A deficiency of testosterone would be obvious if the blood testosterone level was below 8nmol/L, the normal range of testosterone in the blood being 11 to 37nmol/L. This would be further confirmed by high blood levels of the pituitary hormone called Luteinising Hormone (LH), which is indicative that the pituitary gland is trying to stimulate the sluggish testicles. This blood test could be repeated on three separate occasions, and eight-weekly intervals to demonstrate any trends before deciding if male HRT is needed.

The symptoms of testosterone deficiency in men

Testosterone deficiency can produce the following symptoms -
1. Reduced libido
2. Fatigue and behavioural changes
3. Shrinkage (atrophy) of the muscles, testicles and penis and softening of the testicles
4. Reduced rate of growth of facial and body hair
5. Reduction in virility and the ability to achieve orgasm; in severe cases impotence may occur

A male who has previously had high levels of testosterone may find that the decreasing testosterone levels that can begin to occur after the age of 50, produce subtle mental and physical changes, even though his blood test reveals that his testosterone levels are still within the normal physiological range of 11 to 37nmol/L. This is because his testosterone levels are much lower than they used to be and he is sensitive to the decreasing levels.

Subtle changes of decreasing testosterone production may range from depression, loss of confidence, loss of drive and aggression, and loss of competitiveness in all spheres. The warrior man finds himself becoming a bit of a mouse. If such a male takes himself along to the doctor, he may be told that all this is symptomatic of the psychological male midlife crisis, especially after a full physical check-up fails to reveal any medical problems. He may be told that this crisis is due to a plateau in his career, looming retirement, unrealised ambitions, getting older, overdoing it or stress.

He may be offered a course of antidepressants or tranquillisers and referred for counselling to assuage his growing self-doubts. Men are more reluctant than women to accept a course of such therapy, preferring to numb their anxieties at the bar with their mates. Unfortunately, alcohol ingestion, if it becomes regular or excessive, often further reduces the production of testosterone, leading to an aggravation of the mental and physical imbalance. It is vital to check the possibility of a hormonal deficiency and, if this is suspected, a short trial of hormone replacement therapy with testosterone can be tried.

Oral Androgens

The word 'androgen' is the medical term for 'male hormone'.

Androgens may be given on a regular basis in tablet (oral) form. Some common brands are Testomet (methyltestosterone) or Andriol (testosterone undecanoate). There is a possible link between Testomet and liver cancer and Andriol can produce nausea if taken in large doses.

All in all, oral androgens often prove to be unsatisfactory in their effect and a significant proportion of men with severe testosterone deficiency complain that oral testosterone is not effective. It may not be wise to use oral androgens as an introductory trial in a middle-aged man, who has a subtle androgen deficiency and who is wondering whether male hormone replacement therapy holds the key to wellbeing. If oral androgens are ineffectual, a negative value judgement against all other forms of male HRT may be made, with further attempts being rejected.

Androgen Injections

If a man is considering a short-term trial of male HRT, there is probably a no more definitive way of proving or disproving its benefit than with a three month course of monthly injections of androgen. If a deficiency of testosterone is responsible for the mental, physical and sexual fatigue of middle-age, then the androgen injection should greatly reduce, if not abolish, these symptoms within one to two weeks. This brings a great sense of relief and, apart from the alleviation of symptoms, the androgen injections can produce a feeling of great energy, vitality and can be a superb anti-depressant. Suitable androgen injections are Primoteston Depot (testosterone oenanthate) or Sustanon (testosterone propionate), which can be given as a deep oily intramuscular injection into the buttocks each month for three months. A follow-up appointment with the doctor should be made two months after the final injection, by which time their effect would no longer be apparent. During this consultation, a decision to abandon or continue with testosterone replacement therapy in the long term can be made.

Androgen Creams

If a patient decides to continue with testosterone replacement for several years or longer, the safest way to deliver it would be via a hormone cream or patch containing natural testosterone. The cream is rubbed into the skin of the inner upper arm (where there is no hair) once or twice daily after showering. The lowest possible dose of testosterone should be used and many men find that daily doses as small as 5mg are effective in relieving their symptoms.

The adrenal hormone called dehydroepiandrosterone (DHEA) can also be helpful in relieving the symptoms of male menopause and is particularly helpful in chronic fatigue syndrome. The DHEA acts like a weak male hormone and can enhance the effect of testosterone when the two hormones are given together. The DHEA can be added to the testosterone in the same cream. DHEA is available in Australia on a doctor's prescription and doses of DHEA vary from 10 to 50mg daily.

Side effects of androgen replacement therapy

If testosterone and/or DHEA are given in any form, (such as tablets, troches, injections, patches or creams) on a long-term basis, their use needs to be carefully supervised by a doctor. Testosterone replacement therapy, given over several to many years, may cause problems and ideally, the lowest dose of testosterone should be used to maintain a good quality of mental, physical and sexual wellbeing.

Your partner should be made aware that testosterone replacement therapy can increase the size of the prostate gland. The prostate gland is situated at the neck of the bladder and secretes fluid to add to the sperm during ejaculation. If it becomes enlarged, difficulties may be experienced during the passage of urine with such symptoms as difficulty in beginning urination, dribbling after passing urine, slowness and delay in completing urination and urinary frequency occurring. If these problems persist, surgical treatment on the prostate gland may be required. Long-term testosterone replacement therapy may also increase the risk of cancer of the prostate gland. If testosterone doses are excessive, they may produce an unfavourable influence on blood cholesterol patterns thus increasing the risk of cardiovascular disease. Excessive doses may also produce an abnormally high level of red blood cells (polycythaemia).

Overall, testosterone and/or DHEA replacement therapy is safe and can be of tremendous value, provided small doses are used and it is given by an expert in the field and supervised by 6 monthly blood tests and annual checkups from a urologist.

The male mid life crisis

Technically, we know that men cannot go through a literal menopause. However, for many men the phase of midlife brings significant hormonal changes and important physical and psychological changes. Put these all together in a melting pot and you may very well have the ingredients for a male midlife crisis. This is undoubtedly one of the reasons why divorce rates soar at this time and many women get the shock of their lives. These women are left in the well known 'empty nest syndrome' with hubby fleeing the familiar domestic scene. Conversely, the male not infrequently gets the 'nesting syndrome' and spreads his wings with a younger woman, finding that her youthfulness rekindles his feelings of manliness and passion and he feels that life is beginning all over again.

This situation is very emotive and can be extremely traumatic in the short and long term. It could probably be averted in many cases if males received more information and supportive counselling especially with their wives at this time in their lives. In some cases, the timely use of testosterone replacement therapy, even if only on a temporary basis, can bring back the sparkle into a long-term sexual relationship.

If older men keep running of with younger women, what will the women they leave behind do? Well, one obvious strategy is that these women can also get the 'nesting syndrome' and run off with younger men! I see quite a few older women doing this and find it an interesting sociological phenomenon. Anyway, there are statistics to support such behaviour, as women have been found, on average, to live nine to ten years longer than their male counterparts. To avoid loneliness in old age, a man ten years younger could probably fit the bill very nicely!

Nutritional help for a poor libido

Patients often ask me if there is a natural program that they can use to stimulate their flagging libido. Indeed there is and suitable foods to improve the function of your endocrine glands are:

- Seafood especially oysters and cold water fish (salmon, tuna & sardines). Caviar is a well known aphrodisiac and a promoter of fertility. If you cannot afford real caviar, salmon trout eggs will work in the same way. Combined with a ripe avocado it will work even more effectively.

- Legumes such as beans, lentils and peas contain phyto-estrogens to promote hormonal balance

- Raw salads and raw fruits, especially passion fruits

- Free range eggs – six to eight per week

- Raw fruit and vegetable juices are a must

- Whole ground flaxseed provides essential fatty acids which are required for healthy ovarian function.

■ Dark rich chocolate – contains phenylethylamine (PEA), which is a brain chemical (neuro-amine) that reduces depression. Large amounts of PEA naturally flood the nervous system when one falls in love. This is why suitors traditionally offer dark chocolate to their desired lover.

■ Spicy food containing capsicum, hot chillies, cumin, curry, tumeric and coriander will improve the peripheral circulation. The herbs rocket and green coriander have stimulating sexual aromas.

Food as anyone who has taken a prospective lover out to dinner will know - is an important part of fore-play. Nature has inter-twined sex and food with a cascade of pleasure factors designed to promote the continuation of life – a combination of reproduction and nutrition. Aromas and flavours in some foods can act to increase the production of sexually stimulating mental hormones called pheromones. There are five basic human sexual pheromones and the most potent of the pheromones is androstenone; its aroma has been variously described as musk, leather, cedar oil or men's locker rooms. Other aromas that suggest androstenone are truffles, celeri-ac and parsley. Pyrroline is another human pheromone and contributes to the aroma of chestnuts, fresh corn on the cob and persimmons.

Herbal supplements that may help improve libido are:

■ Siberian Ginseng root - this was given to Russian cosmonauts to counteract fatigue, improve muscle stamina and generally boost the endocrine system

■ Horny goat weed is used today to boost the libido, and with a name like that, the power of suggestion should also help anticipation!

■ The herb Tribulus Terrestris has been used for centuries in India for its rejuvenating and aphrodisiacal qualities

■ Gingko biloba improves the peripheral circulation and stamina

■ Muira Puama is grown in South America where it is known as potency wood and enjoys a reputation for increasing sexual stamina and boosting libido. It is still used today as a sexual tonic especially during the festival in Rio.

■ Wild yam which is part of some menopause formulas

These herbs do not give an instant temporary increase in libido but are designed to promote hormonal balance and well being for a sustained effect.

If at first you don't succeed..

What if, after a checkup, hormone replacement therapy and natural supplements, the libido is still flagging? Firstly don't give up prematurely, as it
may be necessary to try several different combinations of hormones and
when the right combination is found, it may take two to three months to
produce the desired effect.

Secondly, take a look at your lifestyle; has it been basically healthy, or are
you drinking and smoking your sex glands into an early death?

Thirdly, take a look at the quality of communication between you and your
partner. Is it blocked by fear, guilt or poor self-image and low self-esteem,
embarrassment, anger, frustration or other negative emotions? If so, you
need to go back to basics and receive some counselling from a professional psychologist or doctor, who has a special interest in sexual disorders.
Such professionals are called sex therapists and this type of counselling
can be combined with counselling from a marriage guidance counsellor, if
necessary. Your local doctor should be able to refer you to these professionals.

It is a rare individual, who will not have some response to these measures.
However, if you cannot rekindle the lost flame of passion and desire,
remember that libido normally has its own biorhythms and you may be in
a temporary natural low.

CHAPTER 12

Polycystic Ovarian Syndrome
by Melissa Nash (B.Sc.Dip.HM) and Dr Cabot

Polycystic Ovarian Syndrome (PCOS) is the most common hormonal problem in women in the reproductive age group; one in every six women probably has the genetic tendency to develop PCOS.

In a normal ovary, a single egg develops and is released from the ovary each month. The release of the egg from the ovary is called ovulation. In Polycystic Ovarian Syndrome (PCOS), normal ovulation is inhibited, and the eggs become trapped in the ovaries. This results in small fluid filled sacs (cysts) in the ovaries.

It is however possible for a woman to have PCOS without actually having the ovarian cysts and in this situation we diagnose it from the symptoms and the blood test results.

PCOS is not a 'new' disease and was originally known as 'Stein and Leventhal Disease' after the doctors that first defined it. They described a group of symptoms that included obesity, hirsutism and infertility in 1935. There have even been mentions made in various writings from hundreds of years ago of 'fat bearded ladies'! These reports have been surmised as being somewhat graphic accounts of unfortunate women with marked cases of PCOS. Since 1935 the story behind the symptoms of PCOS has proven to be even more indepth than what Stein and Levethal could ever have imagined.

The understanding of this syndrome by the medical fraternity is still in its infancy, and until recently it was thought to be fundamentally a gynaecological problem. However, doctors now recognize that the disorder is primarily a hormonal (endocrine) imbalance

What causes the Polycystic Ovarian Syndrome?

PCOS runs in families, so the tendency to develop the syndrome is often inherited.

The exact cause of the hormone imbalance that leads to PCOS is unclear. In some women it is best described as a hormonal imbalance that is set off by insulin resistance and elevated blood levels of insulin. Insulin is a hormone produced by the pancreas gland and its primary function is to regulate the levels of sugar in the blood. How the elevated insulin levels disrupt the body's sex hormone levels, is still not totally understood. The elevated levels of insulin reduce the liver's production of the protein called Sex Hormone Binding Globulin (SHBG). The SHBG binds the body's sex hormones, and if it is reduced, the blood levels of free testosterone become elevated.

Possible symptoms and signs of the Polycystic Ovarian Syndrome

The types of symptoms vary between women and may be found singularly or in combination.

1. Obesity

Up to 70% of patients with PCOS are overweight. Excess weight tends to be centred on the abdominal area.

It is important to note that a significant number of women with PCOS are NOT overweight, and in some cases may be underweight.

One study used ultrasound scans to measure the thickness of the fat just under the skin and also around the internal abdominal organs in non-obese women with PCOS. They compared these measurements with those in non-obese women that did NOT have PCOS. They also measured the levels of hormones, and blood fats (cholesterol and triglycerides) and analysed glucose tolerance and insulin sensitivity. What they discovered was very interesting; the thickness of the subcutaneous fat (which is located just under the skin) was the same in both PCOS and non PCOS subjects, while the deeper hidden layers of fat around the internal organs were significantly thicker in the women with PCOS. The women with PCOS also had a higher incidence of problems with their blood fats (higher triglycerides and total cholesterol, and lower levels of the good HDL cholesterol). These are known markers to increase the risk of cardiovascular disease. (Ref 33)

2. Irregular or absent menstruation

A failure to ovulate regularly presents as a lack of menstrual bleeding in 50% of PCOS patients, and as heavy menstrual bleeding in 30% of patients; however, 20% of PCOS patients will menstruate normally. Some women with PCOS will have irregular infrequent periods and around 20% of women with PCOS have a total absence of menstrual bleeding.

3. Excess levels of male hormones (androgens)

This type of hormonal imbalance occurs in around 70% of women with PCOS and may present as:

Male-pattern hair loss - The hair line tends to recede at the temples and the hair thins at the crown of the head

Hirsutism - Excess hair may be noted on the face, around the nipples and between the navel and pubic area.

Acne and other skin problems - Acne is seen in about 30% of PCOS patients. This is caused by the increased secretion of sebum stimulated by the excess androgens. Skin tags which are lumps of excess skin can form - these are usually found in the armpits or on the neck. Skin discolouration - some women with PCOS have dark patches on the skin around the neck, groin and under the arms. This condition is called acanthosis nigricans and is a sign of insulin resistance (Syndrome X).

4. Infertility

Achieving a spontaneous pregnancy is difficult for many women with PCOS. The presence of the cysts on the ovaries, with no other obvious symptoms, does not definitely signal infertility. In fact studies have shown that women with visible cysts as the sole presenting symptom, have the same fertility rates as women with ovaries of a normal appearance. It is the women that have visible ovarian cysts in conjunction with at least one of the other symptoms associated with PCOS, (such as lack of menstruation, excess androgens or obesity), that usually take longer to fall pregnant. Many women with untreated or uncontrolled PCOS may find conception extremely difficult until they have taken steps to get the hormonal imbalance under control.

If pregnancy is achieved, women with unmanaged PCOS are at a greater risk of problems during pregnancy including gestational diabetes, pregnancy-induced high blood pressure and low birth weight babies.

Clinical signs that the doctor will look for include

1. Ovarian cysts

Most, but not all women with PCOS, have multiple small cysts on their ovaries. An ultrasound scan of the ovaries will show an enlarged ovary with a circlet of small follicles around the outside. Severe cases may have larger multiple cysts.

2. The chemical imbalance of Syndrome X

PCOS is commonly associated with the metabolic disorder called "Syndrome X." Syndrome X is best described as a chemical imbalance that begins with the body becoming resistant to the effects of the hormone insulin. This means that the insulin stops working efficiently, and the body has to compensate by making more and more insulin, and this results in excess levels of insulin. Insulin is a fat storing hormone so that weight gain usually starts to occur, even if the patient is not overeating. Insulin resistance is common in PCOS patients occurring in around 60% of diagnosed cases. If the insulin resistance gets worse, the control of blood sugar levels becomes impaired, and this may lead to raised fasting blood glucose (sugar), elevated blood pressure and eventually type-2 diabetes.

Syndrome X can occur in both obese and lean patients - however it is much worse in women who are overweight. It is often hereditary and is usually aggravated by a high carbohydrate diet. In effect the cells become insensitive to the action of insulin, and so ever greater amounts of insulin are required to keep the blood sugar levels under control. As weight is gained, insulin makes it easier to store fat and harder to lose it. To date, the belief is that insulin resistance occurs mainly in muscle, but is also present in the liver in obese women with PCOS. Some types of cells (most commonly muscle and fat cells) in the body can be insulin resistant, while other types of cells (such as those found in the ovaries, the pituitary gland and adrenal glands) are not insulin resistant. In an insulin resistant patient, these glands will be stimulated by far higher levels of insulin than normal, with the consequences of elevated Luteinising Hormone (LH) and androgens, as seen in patients with PCOS.

The more abdominal fat that a woman has, the more insulin the pancreas will pump out with meals, and the more likely her cells will become resistant to the action of the insulin. Elevated insulin has been shown to stimulate the production of more male hormones from the ovaries, as the ovaries retain their sensitivity to the insulin, even though the muscles and liver do not. Insulin resistance and high levels of insulin are two features of PCOS that are associated with a higher risk of developing Type 2 diabetes later in life.

3. Abnormal blood fats

Women with PCOS tend to have higher levels of LDL cholesterol and triglycerides, which puts them at risk for developing cardiovascular disease. Excess insulin stimulates fat storage and alters cholesterol metabolism, leading to elevated cholesterol and triglyceride levels. Patients will often have high levels of Low-Density Lipoprotein (LDL) or bad cholesterol, and low levels of High-Density Lipoprotein (HDL) or good cholesterol.

4. Imbalances in the levels of sex hormones

Luteinising Hormone (LH) and Follicle Stimulating Hormone (FSH) are made by the pituitary gland and regulate the production of the sex hormones from the ovaries.

In women with PCOS, the LH levels are elevated and the FSH levels stay within the normal range. This is noted in up to 95% of cases if regular menstruation is not occurring, which suggests that this imbalance in LH and FSH levels may be what ultimately causes the lack of ovulation and disruption to the periods.

The levels of LH and FSH are best tested early in the menstrual cycle.

There are three main sex hormones produced in the ovaries - oestrogen, androgen and progesterone. Because ovulation does not occur very often in women with PCOS, adequate amounts of the hormone progesterone will not be produced from the ovaries. However polycystic ovaries do continue to produce oestrogen and androgen, even though ovulation does not occur. The abnormally low progesterone levels prevent the proper development of the fluid filled sac that forms around the egg. Instead, it turns into a cyst in the ovary.

The lack of progesterone may result in -

Absent menstrual periods

Very infrequent menstrual bleeding that can be heavy and/or painful

Reduced fertility

Premenstrual syndrome

An increased risk of the development of uterine (endometrial) cancer

Patients should be monitored for endometrial cancer if they do not have periods or if the periods are very irregular.

The protein called Sex Hormone Binding Globulin (SHBG) is a carrier protein that is made in the liver. SHBG binds the male hormones (androgens) that are floating freely in the blood and renders them 'non-active'. It therefore plays an important role in regulating the amount of 'active' or free male hormone in the body. PCOS sufferers characteristically have elevated levels of free androgens with a low level of SHBG. This is reported in blood tests such as the Free Androgen Index (FAI), which is the ratio of the total male hormones to the SHBG. A high FAI result indicates greater androgen activity in the body, which causes symptoms such as excess facial and body hair, scalp hair loss and acne. Androgens are produced in the ovaries, adrenal glands and also in the upper level body fat. Therefore it is desirable for women with this condition to avoid carrying too much body fat.

Weight excess will aggravate all the hormonal imbalances of the Polycystic Ovarian Syndrome (PCOS) and is often associated with Syndrome X. Women with PCOS have a much higher risk of Syndrome X and a sevenfold increased risk of becoming a Type 2 diabetic, especially if they are overweight. The excess of male hormones will increase insulin resistance so that blood glucose problems, high cholesterol, and hypertension may result, especially in overweight women.

A woman with PCOS may have only one, a few, or all of these symptoms. There are varying degrees of PCOS ranging from severe where a woman suffers from ALL the listed symptoms, to a woman who has ONLY the characteristic ovarian cysts on the ultrasound scan and no other symptoms or signs.

Certain trigger factors can push a woman with very mild PCOS to a more severe expression of symptoms.

The most likely triggers are -

- *Weight excess and weight gain*
- *Excess calorie intake, particularly from highly processed starchy carbohydrate foods*
- *Lack of exercise*
- *Excess intake of male hormones, perhaps from the prescription of oral contraceptive pills, or hormone replacement therapy containing 'masculine' type progesterones.*

Diagnosis of PCOS

Different diagnostic criteria for PCOS are used in different countries. The UK defines PCOS as the appearance of the follicle cysts on an ultrasound scan of the ovaries in combination with one or more of the symptoms already listed. In the US the definition is tighter and requires the combination of irregular periods and excess androgen levels, but does not take into consideration the presence or absence of cysts on the ovaries. So Polycystic Ovarian Syndrome is not automatically diagnosed if cysts on the ovaries are found incidentally when an ultrasound scan is performed, unless one or more of the other signs or symptoms (acne, excess facial hair etc.) are present.

PCOS can be diagnosed by blood tests and an ultrasound scan, which is done with a probe inserted into the vagina (known as a trans-vaginal sonogram). An ultrasound examination of the ovaries is able to visualise the size and shape of the ovaries as well as the cysts.

Physical examination includes a pelvic examination to determine the size of the ovaries, and visual inspection of the skin for hirsutism, acne, or other changes.

A careful evaluation is needed, as it is becoming clear that women who do not suffer from ALL the clinical signs of PCOS may still suffer from all its consequences. Any women that suffers from irregular cycles, lack of menstruation and/or hirsutism should be evaluated for PCOS. Many women with PCOS, especially of a mild degree, remain undiagnosed because the condition is under recognised.

Tests in women with PCOS

To diagnose polycystic ovary syndrome the doctor will perform blood tests to check the hormone levels. Many PCOS patients will have abnormal levels of one or more of these hormones, although normal levels of hormones do not rule out a diagnosis of PCOS. PCOS can be difficult to diagnose since its symptoms are similar to those of other hormonal imbalances, and it can present in a mild or varied form. Doctors face a challenge in diagnosing PCOS, as there is a lack of a solid set of criteria to base a diagnosis on. It is recommended that all women diagnosed with PCOS should have a Glucose Tolerance Test (GGT) with insulin levels, in addition to a fasting blood glucose test. This is because a significant number of women will meet the diagnostic criteria for pre-diabetes or diabetes based on the GTT, although their fasting glucose test registers normal levels. This is the more frightening aspect of this syndrome - the fact that a serious and undiagnosed condition such as diabetes or pre-diabetes, can be slowly brewing over many years, when something could easily be done about it.

Blood tests for hormones should include levels of -

Total testosterone, Free testosterone and Free Androgen Index (FAI)
Oestrogen, SHBG (Sex Hormone Binding Globulin)
LH (Luteinising Hormone), FSH (Follicle Stimulating Hormone)

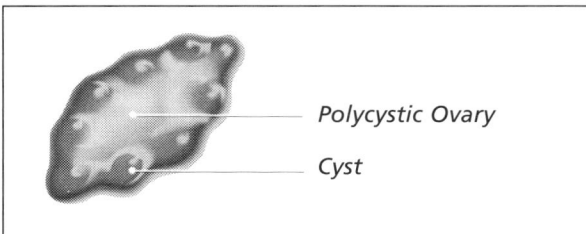

Polycystic Ovary

Cyst

Is PCOS curable?

With proper diagnosis and treatment, most PCOS symptoms can be adequately controlled or eliminated.

Infertility can be corrected and a healthy pregnancy achieved in most patients, although in some, the hormonal disturbances may recur, especially if the patient returns to unhealthy lifestyle and dietary habits and becomes overweight.

The aims of treatment are to -

1. Reduce the levels of fat both from underneath the surface of the skin and around the organs inside the body

2. Reduce elevated insulin levels

3. Improve insulin sensitivity

4. Decrease elevated androgens

5. Reduce the effects of unopposed oestrogen on the uterus

The result of attaining these goals is a reduction in the risk of developing complications such as diabetes, high blood pressure, high cholesterol and uterine cancer.

The mechanisms by which various treatments affect insulin resistance cover a wide spectrum and when it comes to drug prescriptions, there is no one correct way to go about it. This is due to the fact that PCOS can present as many different combinations of symptoms and signs. Studies show differing levels of success when treating the individual symptoms such as hirsutism and insulin resistance with drugs.

Diet

Although insulin-sensitising drugs such as Metformin can help those with PCOS, it is generally agreed that dietary changes remain the best strategy for long term success. The achievement of a normal healthy body weight has been continually shown to be the most effective long term approach in relieving the symptoms of PCOS. In many cases, it is not necessary to lose a lot of weight and it may be possible to regain regular ovulation with as little as an 8% reduction in body fat.

The best diet to follow is one that is low in processed starchy carbohydrate and refined sugars. It can be most effective to avoid all added sugar and all grains such as wheat, rye, barley, oats, rice and corn. Legumes such as beans, peas and lentils are less likely to increase insulin levels and weight gain.

The diet should contain adequate amounts of first class proteins from eggs, seafood, lean fresh meat, low fat cheese, whey protein powder and organic poultry. If you are a vegetarian, first class protein can be obtained by combining legumes, nuts and seeds at the same meal. The diet should be high in vegetables of the raw and cooked variety. Sugar can be replaced with the naturally sweet herb Stevia.

If you are battling with a weight problem you will find the diet in chapter 23 of my book titled *"Can t Lose Weight? You could have Syndrome X"* very effective, for losing your excess weight. This is a low carbohydrate diet and also reduces insulin levels and promotes general well being.

Nutritional Supplements

It is possible to help the body to respond better to the effects of insulin by using nutritional supplements. This will also help you to lose weight. For more information you may phone the Women's Health Advisory Service on 02 4655 8855.

There are specific herbs and nutrients that have been shown to improve glucose and insulin metabolism. They may be taken individually or combined together in some formulas for a synergistic effect.

The most effective are a combination of the following-

Gymnema Sylvestre (GS)

According to several human clinical trials, the action of the herb Gymnema Sylvestre can be beneficial in those with elevated blood glucose levels. High blood levels of glucose (hyperglycaemia), high cholesterol and excessive glycosylation of proteins, which are associated with insulin resistance, are improved by Gymnema Sylvestre. Gymnema also reduces cravings for sugar and refined carbohydrates. Clinical trials of Gymnema Sylvestre used an equivalent of 400mg daily of the whole herb from a 5:1 extract of Gymnema Sylvestre.

Bitter Melon

The herb Bitter Melon is also known as Momordica Charantia, or Bitter Gourd. The fruit of this plant, which is a member of the Cucurbitaceae family, is a popular food in India. Clinical trials and laboratory experiments using an extract of the dried fruit or ground seeds of Bitter Melon, revealed its ability to lower blood glucose levels. These studies found that Bitter Melon reduces blood glucose levels and improves glucose tolerance in Type 2 diabetics. It is able to reduce blood glucose levels, thus reducing the need for high insulin output. The recommended daily dosage of Bitter Melon is an equivalent of 5 grams of the fruit powder using an 8:1 standardised extract. (Ref 34)

Chromium picolinate

The mineral chromium is required for the healthy function of the insulin receptors, which are situated on the surface of the cells. This is very important for those with insulin resistance where the receptors malfunction, and become resistant to the action of insulin. In other words chromium helps the cells to communicate better with the insulin hormone, thereby facilitating the transfer of glucose from the blood stream into the cell to be used as cellular energy. Deficiency of chromium is common in those who have consumed a diet high in refined carbohydrates. In those with Syndrome X, I highly recommend a supplement, which contains chromium picolinate. It is difficult to get all the chromium you need from your diet, as the richest sources are Brewer s yeast and liver. Chromium is a vital component of Glucose Tolerance Factor (GTF), which improves insulin function. Those who are deficient in chromium have difficulty in regulating blood glucose levels. Chromium deficiency may be associated with anxiety, fatigue, sugar cravings, excess hunger, glucose intolerance and high cholesterol. Many people who supplement with chromium picolinate find that their craving for carbohydrates and sweets diminishes greatly. There have also been reports that chromium supplements can help the conversion of excess body fat into lean muscle tissue.

Chromium picolinate has been shown to reduce insulin resistance, and lower blood glucose levels by 18%. (Ref 35)

Lipoic Acid

Lipoic acid is a natural substance, which has been demonstrated to be effective in improving glucose utilization, which is critical to managing those with Syndrome X or diabetes. Supplementation with lipoic acid provides substantial health benefits to those with Syndrome X; doses of lipoic acid range from 100 to 600mg daily. (Ref 36)

Carnitine fumarate

Carnitine is a natural substance made in the human body from the essential amino acids lysine and methionine. Carnitine is involved in fat mobilisation, and when it is deficient, overweight persons often find it very difficult to get into the fat burning area of metabolism. In other words, they have difficulty beginning the breakdown of body fat, which is called the stage of lipolysis and ketosis. Supplemental carnitine may increase the burn rate of calories from stored fat by enhancing the efficiency of fatty acid oxidation. The richest dietary sources of carnitine are red meats (lamb and beef). Vegetables, fruits and many cereals contain little or no carnitine.

Selenium

Selenium should be supplemented in those with Syndrome X, and in diabetics, because of its proven protective effects on cell membranes and genetic material. (Ref 37)

Synergistic Minerals

Magnesium, manganese and zinc are involved in multiple enzyme systems within the energy producing mitochondria. A diet high in carbohydrates, especially of the refined types, may cause depletion of minerals such as magnesium, manganese, selenium and zinc, which will have an adverse effect upon the immune system, and slow down metabolism.

A low magnesium level has been associated with insulin resistance, high levels of insulin and blood glucose abnormalities. Magnesium has been shown to reduce insulin resistance and I highly recommend that you take supplemental magnesium if you have Syndrome X

Trace mineral deficiencies are not uncommon in those with Syndrome X, and may worsen glucose intolerance.

The nutrients discussed above are helpful for -

Insulin resistance and insulin excess = Syndrome X

Unstable blood glucose levels including high blood glucose levels (hyperglycaemia) and low blood glucose levels (hypoglycaemia)

Cravings for sugar and high GI carbohydrates

Weight excess in those with impaired glucose tolerance

For more information on nutritional supplements and diet for PCOS you may call the Health Advisory Service on 02 4655 8855

Exercise

Studies have shown that exercise programs that specifically combine aerobic exercise (such as jogging, walking and swimming) along with a resistance program (such as low impact exercise with weights) will improve insulin sensitivity. It seems that the effects last for around 3 to 6 days after the last exercise session. Therefore, exercise is recommended at least three times per week, to get the maximum long term benefit.

Orthodox Treatment

Metformin

Metformin is a drug which acts by-

Decreasing the liver's production of glucose

Decreasing the intestinal absorption of glucose

Improving insulin sensitivity

Metformin has been shown in some studies to have a beneficial effect on menstrual regulation and has shown promising results in PCOS patients with hirsutism, but its effects on infertility and other PCOS symptoms are unknown. Drug treatment of hirsutism is long-term, and improvement may not be seen for up to a year or longer. Whether the addition of insulin sensitizing drugs like Metformin to healthy diet and lifestyle changes, is of significant benefit, is still under debate.

Hormone balancing

Natural progesterone

Most women with PCOS are deficient in progesterone. Many of these patients can benefit from the use of natural progesterone in the form of creams, troches or capsules. Natural progesterone does not aggravate insulin resistance or cholesterol problems, whereas synthetic progestogens do. Natural progesterone does not increase weight, and may help to relieve many of the symptoms of PCOS. The use of natural progesterone will confer a protective effect on the lining of the uterus (endometrium) and thus reduce the risk of uterine cancer. Natural progesterone does not provide contraception and may increase fertility. For more information on progesterone see page 29

The oral contraceptive pill (OCP)

Most women diagnosed with PCOS will be put on the OCP to produce a regular menstrual bleed. The OCP can prevent the overgrowth of the uterine lining (endometrium) associated with progesterone deficiency; however natural progesterone can achieve the same benefit. Unlike natural progesterone, the OCP does provide effective contraception. However, the choice of OCP is very important. Many OCPs on the market contain masculinised synthetic progestogens that actually worsen the excess androgen component of PCOS. Progestogens that are best avoided include norethisterone, norgestrel, and levonorgestrel because they are particularly androgenic. These androgenic progestogens will also worsen the other aspects of PCOS, such as insulin resistance and weight gain in some women.

Drospirenone is a new age progestogen that has anti-androgenic activities - it is combined with synthetic oestrogen in the brand of the OCP called Yasmin and is useful in managing the symptoms of PCOS - for more information on Yasmin see page 88

Other suitable feminine brands of the OCP for women with PCOS are Diane, Brenda, Juliet, Femoden, Minulet and Marvelon.

Anti male hormones (anti-androgens)

These drugs act by reducing the body's production of androgens, interfering with the action of the androgens and/or increasing the production of the binding protein called Sex Hormone Binding Globulin (SHBG). Anti-androgen drugs may be used when androgenic symptoms (such as facial hair, excess body hair, balding and acne) are unresponsive to body fat reduction or oral contraceptive pills. It is vital that pregnancy is avoided when taking anti-androgen medications, as these can have a feminising effect on a male foetus. It is for this reason that anti-androgens are usually combined with, or are part of the OCP.

Examples of anti-androgens are -

Cyproterone acetate

This drug acts by inhibiting the binding of androgens to receptors on the cell and is a very effective treatment for acne, male pattern baldness and hirsutism. For more information on cyproterone see page 125.

Spironolactone (Aldactone)

This drug may be given alone or with an oral contraceptive pill and improves hirsutism, acne and male-pattern baldness. It has no effect on fertility. Spironolactone is not as effective as cyproterone. Spironolactone may cause abnormal uterine bleeding and is linked with birth defects if taken during pregnancy. For more information see page 126

Flutamide (Eulexin)

This drug has the effect of reducing the amount of fat surrounding the abdominal organs (visceral fat) and reduces hirsutism. It also reduces the levels of the androgenic hormones and reduces Low Density Lipoprotein (LDL) cholesterol. However, flutamide is expensive and can cause liver abnormalities, fatigue, mood swings, and loss of sexual desire.

GnRH Agonists

Some patients have severe hirsutism that does not respond to diet, OCPs or anti-androgens. These women may be given monthly injections for six months of a synthetic version of a hormone produced in the brain called GnRH. This chemically 'turns off' the ovaries and induces a medical menopause. The result is a great reduction in the amount of androgens produced by the ovaries.

GnRH Agonist drugs can only be given for 6 months, as they increase the risk of osteoporosis and would only be considered as a last resort after all other approaches have failed.

Thankfully the majority of patients will respond very favourably to diet, exercise, nutritional supplementation and hormone balancing.

Fertility and pregnancy

A drug that helps to trigger ovulation is the steroid hormone dexamethasone. This drug acts by reducing the production of androgens by the adrenal glands. This condition is best evaluated by a reproductive endocrinologist, rather than an obstetrician-gynaecologist or regular endocrinologist.

If an infertile patient desires pregnancy, the first drug usually given to help induce ovulation is clomiphene citrate (Clomid). Clomid results in pregnancy in about 70% of patients but does increase the risk of multiple births. In the 25% of women who do not respond to Clomid, other drugs that stimulate follicle development and induce ovulation can be tried. These include human menopausal gonadotropin (Pergonal) and human chorionic gonadotropin (HCG), and these drugs have a lower pregnancy rate (less than 30%), a higher rate of multiple pregnancy (from 5-30%, depending on the dose of the drug), and a higher risk of medical problems.

PCOS patients have a high rate of miscarriage (30%), and may be treated with the gonadotropin-releasing hormone agonist leuprolide (Lupron) or luteal support agents such as progesterone to reduce this risk.

About Melissa Nash

Melissa Nash B.Sc.Dip.HM is a clinical nutritionist who has been working closely with Dr Cabot for seven years. She has a particular interest in diet and weight and the effects these have on liver health and reproductive disorders - in particular Polycystic Ovarian Syndrome. Melissa suffered with PCOS for many years until she learnt to manage it successfully with diet, supplementation and exercise. Melissa is currently undertaking Post Graduate studies in Biomedical Science. Melissa is available for consultation at Dr Cabot's Broadway Clinic and is also online at www.whas.com.au and www.weightcontroldoctor.com

Chapter 13

Infertility

Couples are considered normally fertile if they achieve a pregnancy within 2 years of regular sexual intercourse. Statistics show that around 85% of couples will conceive in the first year and around 93% by 2 years. Around 15% of couples will have difficulty in conceiving during their fertile years and 10 to 12% will be infertile.

Causes of Infertility

The causes of infertility may be found in only the female or the male, or there may be causes in both sexes. Generally speaking the causes of infertility occur equally in both sexes. Even after extensive investigation it will not be possible to find any definitive cause for the infertility in around 18 to 25% of infertile couples. This is called "unexplained infertility." In the future new research developments will allow us to discover and treat some of the currently unexplained causes of infertility.

Let us look at the known causes of infertility

Female Factors

1. Problems with ovulation

Around 20% of infertile women have problems with ovulation. This is evident because they do not have regular menstrual bleeding and may have very irregular or absent bleeding.

The causes of impaired ovulation are-

Polycystic Ovarian Syndrome (see page 153)
Dysfunction of the hypothalamus-pituitary communication in the brain
High levels of prolactin production from the pituitary gland
Weight excess or very low body weight
Extreme sports activity
Ageing ovaries with poor quality of the ovarian eggs
Genetic chromosomal defects
Prolonged or severe stress

2. Progesterone Deficiency

The production of progesterone from the ovary can only occur if ovulation occurs. Women who do not ovulate will not produce any progesterone.

Progesterone is the hormone of fertility and is produced from the corpus luteum gland in the ovary after ovulation. Progesterone prepares the lining of the uterus (the endometrium) so that it is ready to accept implantation and growth of the fertilised egg. If there is a deficiency of progesterone, the fertilised egg will find the lining of the uterus inhospitable and unsuitable for its implantation. Thus growth and development of the embryo will not occur properly and a miscarriage will be likely to occur. This may happen very early, so that a woman never even realises that she was pregnant, or may occur later sometime during the first 3 months of the pregnancy.

Progesterone deficiency may occur for the following reasons

Stress may upset the pituitary messages to the ovary which make the ovary produce progesterone

Nutritional deficiencies may cause the production of progesterone to be inadequate

Poor circulation of blood to the ovary

Ageing eggs may not have the ability to produce adequate progesterone

3. Non-hormonal causes of Infertility

Endometriosis

This is caused by the growth of the cells which are normally confined within the uterine lining (endometrium) in abnormal places, outside of the uterus. These cells take root in the pelvic and abdominal cavity and grow on the surface of organs such as the bladder, the bowel and the ovaries. They act like a "weed" and continue to grow, and under the influence of the pituitary hormones, these cells will shed and cause internal bleeding, which may block the fallopian tubes and damage the ovaries. This abnormally sited tissue can cause a lot of scarring and inflammation, which will impair the ability of the egg to travel from the ovaries into the fallopian tubes. The tubes may become twisted, scarred and blocked by the abnormal endometrial tissue. Endometriosis often causes severe period pains, heavy bleeding and painful intercourse, however it can also exist in a mild form and not produce any obvious symptoms. It is diagnosed by laparoscopic examination by a gynaecologist.

Problems with the fallopian tubes

The fallopian tubes must be patent and reasonably healthy to allow the egg to be fertilised within them and also to allow the egg to travel through the tube into the uterine cavity where it will implant into the uterine lining. The fallopian tubes can become blocked, scarred and twisted by –

- Endometriosis
- Pelvic infections and inflammation
- Previous abdominal/pelvic surgery, which results in scar tissue on the tubes

Problems with the uterine lining

The endometrium may be too thin because of nutritional deficiencies or previous curettage. It may also be chronically inflamed and scarred from pelvic and genital infections. The endometrium may be distorted by large fibroid tumours in the muscle of the uterus.

Problems with the cervix

The cervix may be scarred and blocked from previous infection or surgery. The mucous production from the cervix and the vagina may be inadequate, or the mucus may be hostile to the sperm. Some women have antibodies in their cervical mucus which attacks the sperm.

Male Factors

Sperm abnormalities

There may be a deficient quantity of sperm and/or the quality of the sperm may be defective. There may be impaired mobility of the sperm so that they are unable to travel all the way into the fallopian tubes.

The can be due to –
- Nutritional deficiencies
- Poor diet and lifestyle
- Stress
- Exposure to toxic chemicals
- Some medications or previous chemotherapy
- Chronic infections in the testes or its tubes

The effect on fertility of advancing age

The negative effect on fertility of getting older, especially in women, is often underestimated by infertile couples.

Natural fertility rates, as well as the success rates of assisted reproduction, start to decline in women reaching their mid-30s. Fertility rates then reduce further in women over 40, and generally speaking, around 30 to 40% of couples, where the women is aged over 39, will have some difficulty with fertility. This is due to the fact that the rate of loss of eggs from the ovaries accelerates during the 10 to 15 years before the menopause. Most women are unaware of this and they assume that if they do not have menopausal symptoms, their ovaries must still be working efficiently. Older women should be referred for investigation of infertility as soon as possible, as they have less time to experiment.

Investigation of the Infertile Couple

It is always important to assess both partners of the infertile couple

Tests in the Female

Hormone levels

1. Progesterone

Blood Progesterone levels should be checked after ovulation – usually seven days before the next expected period. It can be difficult to pinpoint the exact time when progesterone levels should be highest, which is seven days after ovulation. The use of salivary levels of progesterone can be done daily after ovulation right up to the beginning of the period, and this will give a better overall picture of progesterone production. Ideally one should do blood and salivary levels of progesterone, as it is such an important hormone for fertility.

2. Follicle Stimulating Hormone (FSH) and Luteinising Hormone (LH)

FSH and LH are hormones that are produced from the pituitary gland to stimulate the development and ovulation of the ovarian egg. If the levels of FSH and LH are persistently elevated, it means that the ovaries are starting to fail. This can be due to depletion of eggs from the ovary or resistant ovaries which will not respond to the FSH and LH.

3. Male hormones (androgens) and Sex Hormone Binding Globulin (SHBG).

The best way to measure the total active androgens in the body is with the blood test called the Free Androgen Index (FAI). The FAI will be elevated in women with Polycystic Ovarian Syndrome and Syndrome X induced-obesity. These are common causes of infertility and will be associated with lowered levels of SHBG.

4. Thyroid hormone levels

Thyroid gland problems such as over-active or under-active thyroid function, and high levels of antibodies against the thyroid gland can impair fertility. In general these problems are easily rectified with a normalisation of fertility.

5. Prolactin hormone levels

If blood tests reveal abnormally high levels of prolactin there will be reduced ovarian function and fertility will be impaired.

Other tests which may be required are

A pelvic ultrasound scan – this is to check the anatomy and function of the uterus and ovaries. The transvaginal ultrasound technique is very helpful.
Hysteroscopy and laparoscopy to visualise the uterus, tubes, ovaries and pelvic cavity
Analysis of the sperm (semen analysis)
Testing the cervical mucous for the presence of anti-sperm antibodies
Testing the compatibility of the cervical/vaginal mucus with the sperm

Hormonal treatment of Infertility

Inducing Ovulation

This is used for women whose ovaries do not ovulate regularly, such as those with Polycystic Ovarian Syndrome or resistant ovaries. It is not as effective for older women whose ovaries no longer have adequate numbers of good quality eggs to respond to the ovulation stimulating drugs.

The drugs used to stimulate ovulation are

■ Clomiphene – this is the most popular drug used, and produces very good results provided there is no significant problem with the hypothalamus

■ Gonadotrophins –these are given by injection

If these drugs are used by an expert in infertility treatments and their effects are closely monitored, the risk of multiple pregnancies can be kept below 10%.

In many overweight women with unexplained infertility it is possible to induce natural ovulation simply with weight loss and often only a small to moderate weight loss is required. Weight excess is often associated with high levels of insulin, which switch off the ovaries, and this is seen most often in women with polycystic ovarian syndrome. Weight loss causes the excess levels of insulin to reduce and the ovaries come to life again and ovulation recommences spontaneously. This is a welcome relief to women who otherwise face the prospect of having to use drugs to stimulate ovulation. I recommend that if you are overweight you try to lose weight first before trying the ovulation stimulating drugs or even invitro fertilisation. This is because if you become pregnant while significantly overweight, you have a greater chance of complications during pregnancy such as miscarriage and diabetes of pregnancy (gestational diabetes).

Body toxicity and/or fatty liver are often associated with weight excess and reduced ability to ovulate regularly. This was obvious in the case of a 45 year old Japanese woman who had been infertile for 5 years whom I met in Los Angeles. This woman had a fatty liver, which caused her liver enzymes to become elevated and made it impossible for her to lose weight. This woman used my Syndrome X eating plan (see chapter 23 of my book titled *"Cant Lose Weight? You could have Syndrome X"* and took a liver tonic, which resulted in weight loss of 20 kilograms and normalisation of her liver enzymes. She ovulated spontaneously within 6 months and conceived, and had a healthy pregnancy with a normal delivery of a healthy girl. I had the pleasure of meeting her with her beautiful 6 month old baby girl who looked like a happy little Japanese doll. Understandably she and her husband were delighted. So even at the age of 45, fertility is greatly improved with normalisation of body weight and improvement of liver function.

In some women a detoxification program using a liver cleansing diet, raw juicing and a liver tonic can increase fertility. See www.liverdoctor.com. This is because fat-soluble toxins derived from petrochemicals can lodge themselves in the liver (especially if it is fatty) and in the ovaries, which are also fatty organs. These toxic chemicals can disrupt the function of the ovaries impairing regular ovulation and fertility. Thus a detox and liver-cleansing program can work wonders for fertility. If you believe that you have been exposed to a high load of toxic environmental and/or dietary chemicals I recommend that you start to use organic produce, increase your water intake and use a water purifier. Culinary seaweeds such as arame, wakame and dulse can help to rid the body of heavy metal poisons and I recommend that you source organic seaweeds from the health food store.

Progesterone

In a significant number of women with reduced fertility of unexplained origin, there is a deficiency of progesterone production from the ovaries during the latter 2 weeks of the menstrual cycle. Progesterone levels can be assessed with blood and/or salivary tests, and the best time to measure the progesterone is around day 21 of the cycle, which is 7 days before the expected onset of menstrual bleeding. If the progesterone levels are abnormally low, it can be most worthwhile to administer natural progesterone during the last 2 weeks of the cycle. The progesterone can be continued during the first few weeks of the pregnancy to supplement the ovarian production of progesterone. By increasing progesterone levels we can improve the ability of the fertilised egg to implant and grow successfully in the uterine lining.

The use of natural progesterone may be very effective for women who have a problem with very early recurrent miscarriages.

Progesterone can also be worth trying in women with so called "unexplained infertility"

Doses vary between 100 to 400 mg daily, and progesterone can be given in the form of a transdermal or vaginal cream or a troche (lozenge). You need a doctor's prescription for natural progesterone.

In the context of unexplained infertility I think that progesterone is a very underestimated and under used hormone.

Nutritional medicine to improve fertility

The quality of the sperm can be greatly increased with an improvement in diet and lifestyle. Similarly the health of the female reproductive organs and the production of the fertility hormones can be greatly improved with nutritional medicine. Avoid toxins such as cigarettes, excess alcohol, pesticides and industrial chemicals.

When trying to improve fertility I recommend

- A diet high in raw fruits and vegetables
- An intake of first class protein three times daily - this can be achieved from lean fresh red and white meats, organic chicken, eggs, any seafood, or by combining legumes, nuts, grains and seeds at the same meal
- Raw juicing can improve fertility by helping the liver and immune system. Raw juicing using vegetables of many different colours, including dark leafy greens, will boost the intake of the fertility nutrient folic acid

Supplements to increase fertility

- Essential fatty acids (from cold pressed oils, especially flaxseed oil, oily fish, raw seeds, raw nuts and avocados) are vital for healthy ovarian function.
- Vitamin E, the fertility properties of which the ancient Greeks recognised so much, that they named it "tocopherol" meaning the nutrient of fertility.

- Vitamin C to protect the sperm and ovarian eggs and citrus juices and capsicum are excellent source of this fertility vitamin.
- Selenium and zinc are essential for healthy eggs and sperm.
- Folic acid can improve fertility and also reduces the incidence of birth defects in the baby.
- Vitamin B 12 should be supplemented in women who are strict veg ans (those who do not eat any meat, seafood, eggs or dairy products)

If blood tests reveal low levels of iron, it is vital to take an iron supplement. The absorption of iron supplements can be improved by taking them with citrus fruits or vitamin C.

Millions of women suffer from hormonal imbalances from younger women traumatised by acne and pre-menstrual syndrome, to mothers struggling with postnatal depression, to grandmothers, whose well-deserved rest is broken by attacks of hot flushes. Hormonal upheavals can often be blamed for recurring headaches, sexual dysfunction, problems after hysterectomy and tubal ligation, unwanted hair, balding, chronic fatigue and general poor health. In the 1980s, we discovered the vital link between oestrogen deficiency and the epidemic of osteoporosis and cardiovascular disease that cripples our ageing female population.

The majority of women have coped admirably with such hormonal problems but, in a significant minority, these problems have had ruinous effects resulting in severe depression, family disruption, child battering, loss of self-esteem, drug addiction and even suicide. It can be very frightening to feel a victim of one's hormones, knowing that month after month unpleasant symptoms will recur to remind us of our uniquely female vulnerability.

When we understand that the hormonal system of a woman is such a delicate and complex network of interacting body chemicals, it is not surprising that, at times, it seems to go haywire! Not only are we vulnerable to our hormonal fluctuations but our hormones are influenced by our weight, lifestyle, exercise patterns, stress, diet, nutritional imbalances and increasing age.

To fine-tune our hormones is obviously a very specialised and complicated endeavour. It is now possible for the first time in history to achieve this because of new breakthroughs in the speciality of women's hormones (Gynaecological Endocrinology).

Thankfully the attitude of society and doctors towards women with hormonal problems is changing. These problems have their hilarious side as depicted by the cartoons in this book and they also have their tragic side with a propensity to devastate the lives of many women. Doctors are finally realising that women with hormonal problems want to be taken seriously and offered real and lasting solutions. They don't want to be stereotyped, patronised, trivialised or kept in the dark. It does not help to be told that your symptoms are inevitable, a natural part of womanhood or just a sign of your age.

I have written this book because, every day I am challenged with women, whose lives are being turned upside down by their hormones. These women are not neurotic or inadequate. They are intelligent, articulate, strong and very relatable personalities. They recognise that powerful hormonal forces are causing mental and/or physical changes that they need help to control so that their lives can be productive, fulfilled and stable.

I, myself, have had to find solutions for my own hormonally caused health problems that were preventing me from enjoying my life and 'getting on with it', so to speak. Thus I know how it feels to be a victim of one's hormones and thankfully, I now know how to gain control over my own hormonal demons. To have overcome these horrible symptoms in myself and many of my patients, has given me great satisfaction, understanding and compassion.

I hope that this book enables me to share my many years of accumulated clinical research and experience with you. This book *"Hormones - Don't Let them Ruin Your Life"* aims to give you more insight and to show you all your treatment options with an emphasis on natural hormone and nutritional therapies. It is designed to give you the tools that you will need to work with your doctor in conquering the many hormonal problems that may befall you.

APPENDIX - Blood Test Results

This table shows the normal blood levels of the female sex hormones. Their levels fluctuate during the different phases of the normal monthly menstrual cycle and that is why the normal ranges are wide.

TIMING DURING MONTHLY CYCLE	OESTROGEN (as oestradiol) Units = pmol/L	PROGESTERONE Units = nmol/L	FSH Units = IU/L	LH Units = IU/L
Basal			2 – 10	
Follicular	130 - 620	0.1 – 4.3	2 - 12	2 - 12
Peri-ovulatory & mid-cycle	500 - 2000	0.1 – 19.9	9 - 30	Less than 15
Luteal		5.8 - 96		
Mid-Luteal	290 - 1400	16.4 - 117	2 - 12	2 - 15
Post-Menopausal	Less than 150	Less than 2.5	Over 25	Greater than 10
Pre-puberty	Less than 73	Less than 2.5	Less than 6	Less than 4

Explanation notes for table above
Interpretation of blood progesterone levels
• Less than 7 = no ovulation
• Between 7 and 25 = possible ovulation
• Greater than 25 = probable ovulation

The tables below show the normal ranges in the blood of other hormones in women.

Explanation notes for the tables below
The Free Androgen Index (FAI) is calculated in the laboratory by expressing the testosterone amount as a percentage of the SHBG value. The FAI gives a measurement of the amount of free and thus active testosterone in the body.

Hormone	Total testosterone Units = nmol/L	Free testosterone Units = pmol/L	Free Androgen Index (FAI) As a %
Values of the normal range	1.0 - 4.6	Less than 7.0	1.0 – 8.0

Hormone	Prolactin Units = mIU/L	Sex Hormone Binding Globulin (SHBG) Units = nmol/L	Dehydro-epiandrosterone (DHEAS) Units = umol/L
Values of the normal range	40 - 570	30 - 90	Pre-menopause 1.8 -12.0 Post-menopause 0.3 – 1.6 Pre-puberty 0.3 – 1.5

Reference Ranges of hormones measured in the saliva

HORMONE	FEMALE FOLLICULAR	FEMALE LUTEAL	POST- MENOPAUSAL
Oestradiol	2-10 pmol/L	6-14 pmol/L	2-8 pmol/L
Progesterone	50-200 pmol/L	140-520 pmol/L	50-200 pmol/L

HORMONE	FEMALE	MALE
Testosterone	25-190 pmol/L	100-400 pmol/L
DHEA-S	2.5-25 nmol/L	5.0-30 nmol/L

Notes for the tables above

The follicular phase is the first half of the menstrual cycle, before ovulation occurs, in a premenopausal woman.

The luteal phase is the second half of the menstrual cycle, after ovulation occurs, in a premenopausal woman.

After menopause, ovulation ceases, and so these phases of the menstrual cycle become non-existent. During the post-menopause, the natural hormone levels remain at consistently low levels, unless HRT is given.

Scientific references for salivary hormone testing are available on the web site www.arlaus.com.au, which can help patients to understand their salivary test results more easily.

ADRENAL GLANDS - Two small glands sited on top of the kidneys, which secrete steroid hormones and the stress hormone adrenalin.

AIDS - Acquired Immune Deficiency Syndrome

ALOPECIA - Abnormal and excessive loss of hair.

AMENORRHOEA - An abnormal absence of menstrual bleeding.

ANABOLIC STEROIDS - Male hormones, which stimulate the growth of bone, muscle, and body and facial hair.

ANDROGEN - Male hormone

ANDROGENIC - Having a masculine effect and thus stimulating growth of hair in a male pattern, oily skin, deepening of the voice and increased muscle mass.

ANTI-MALE HORMONE - A hormone, which blocks the synthesis and effects of male hormones and is capable of reversing masculine body features.

ANTIOXIDANT - Substances such as vitamins A, C and E, beta-carotene and selenium, which protect the cellular structures from oxidative damage caused by free radicals.

ATROPHY - Wasting or thinning of tissues or organs.

BENIGN - Non-cancerous or non-malignant.

BIOFLAVONOIDS - Bioflavonoids, sometimes referred to as vitamin P, are found in plants along with vitamin C and exert a beneficial effect upon the walls of the blood and lymphatic vessels. This is very helpful for women troubled with fluid retention and puffy limbs.

BODY MASS INDEX (BMI) - The BMI is a scientific way of examining 'fatness' and 'thinness' and is worked out according to the formula: BMI = weight (kilogram)/height squared (metres^2). The normal BMI ranges from 20 to 25 kg/m^2 and many hormonal and menstrual problems can be overcome by keeping weight in the normal BMI range.

BODY TYPE - There are four body shapes or physiques, namely Gynaeoid, Thyroid, Android and Lymphatic. (see www.weightcontroldoctor.com)

BREAKTHROUGH BLEEDING - Irregular vaginal bleeding or spotting occurring in women when they are on the OCP or HRT

CANCER - A malignant growth/tumour with rapid multiplication of abnormal cells that may spread to and invade distant body parts.

CARDIOVASCULAR DISEASE - Disease of the system of the blood circulation comprising the heart and blood vessels.

CAT SCAN - A computerised x-ray of consecutive sections of the body.

CELLULITE - Fatty deposits resulting in a dimply or lumpy appearance of the skin, which is difficult to remove with diet and exercise.

CERVIX - The lower part of the uterus projecting down into the vagina. It is also called the mouth of the womb.

CHLOASMA - Brownish pigmentation of the face caused by some types of hormone therapy and pregnancy.

CHOLESTEROL - A constituent of all animal fats and oils. It is found in the blood in two forms: 1. High Density Lipo-Protein (HDL), which protects against atherosclerosis; 2. Low Density Lipo-Protein, which promotes atherosclerosis.

CLITORIS - The female equivalent of the penis. It is a small bulb found at the top of the vulva, just below the pubic bone and is covered by a hood of tissue. It contains erectile tissue, which is very sensitive to stimulation and adds greatly to a woman's sexual excitement.

CLUSTER HEADACHE - A severe and intense headache, which lasts several hours and may recur frequently over a six to eight week period.

COMBINED ORAL CONTRACEPTIVE PILL - A contraceptive pill containing both female sex hormones, oestrogen and progesterone.

CONCEPTION - The fertilisation of the female egg by the spermatozoa.

CONTRA-INDICATION - A medical condition that makes it inadvisable to use a certain medication, eg the presence of blood clots would contra-indicate the use of the contraceptive pill.

CORPUS LUTEUM - The yellow coloured gland, which is formed within the ovary from the remains of the follicle after it has released its contained egg at ovulation. The corpus luteum manufacturers the hormone progesterone.

CORTISOL - A steroid hormone made by the adrenal glands and also synthetically in laboratories. It improves well-being and has a powerful anti-inflammatory effect.

CUSHING'S SYNDROME - A collection of symptoms and signs, such as a moon-shaped face, buffalo hump and high blood pressure caused by excessive amounts of cortisone.

CYSTIC ACNE - A skin disorder manifesting as blocked pores and pimples, many of which are blind cysts containing pus. It is a severe form of acne.

DIATHERMY   - The surgical technique of burning tissues with a controlled electric current.

DIURETIC - A substance, whether synthetic or natural, which stimulates the kidneys to excrete salt (sodium chloride) and water, thereby relieving fluid retention.

ECTOPIC PREGNANCY - A pregnancy growing in an abnormal position, usually inside a fallopian tube.

ENDOCRINE GLANDS - Glands that manufacture and secrete hormones.

ENDOCRINOLOGIST - A medical specialist in diseases of the endocrine glands and their hormones.

ENDOCRINOLOGY - The study and treatment of disorders of the glands and the hormones they secrete.

ENDOMETRIOSIS - The presence of endometrium (which is normally confined inside the uterine cavity) outside of the uterus scattered about inside the abdomen and pelvic cavities.

ENZYMES - Proteins produced by living cells, which function as catalysts in specific biochemical reactions.

ESSENTIAL FATTY ACIDS - Fatty acids necessary for cellular metabolism, which cannot be made by the body but must be supplied in the diet. Suitable sources are oil of evening primrose, flaxseed oil, fish, fish oil, nuts, seeds and their oils.

FALLOPIAN TUBES - The tubes, which carry the egg (ovum) from the ovary to the uterus. Fertilisation of the egg occurs in the outer part of the fallopian tube.

FEMALE SEX HORMONES - The two sex hormones produced by the female ovary - namely oestrogen and progesterone.

FERTILISATION - The union of the female egg (ovum) with the male egg (spermatozoa) which occurs in the fallopian tube.

FIBROIDS - Non-cancerous growths of the uterus, consisting of muscle and fibrous tissue.

FOETUS - A developing human.

FOLLICLE STIMULATING HORMONE (FSH) - A hormone secreted by the pituitary gland, which reaches the ovaries via the blood circulation and stimulates the growth of ovarian follicles (eggs).

'FRIENDLY PROGESTERONES' - Those types of progesterone that exert a favourable effect upon our blood vessels and skin and do not increase cholesterol, promote weight gain or masculine changes in the skin. Examples are cyproterone acetate, gestodene or desogestrel.

GALACTORRHOEA - The discharge of milk or milky fluid from the nipples when not breast-feeding; inappropriate lactation.

GLANDS - Organs or tissues, generally soft and fleshy in consistency, that manufacture and secrete, or excrete, hormones that exert their effect elsewhere in the body.

GYNAECOLOGY - Study of diseases of women.

GYNAECOLOGICAL ENDOCRINOLOGY - Study of hormones produced by women. It is a relatively new medical speciality, which is expanding rapidly and brings the promise of exciting new developments and hope for many women.

HIRSUTISM - A condition of excessive facial and body hair, excluding the scalp.

HORMONES - Chemicals produced by various glands, which are then transported around the body.

HORMONE REPLACEMENT THERAPY (HRT) - The administration of hormonal preparations (natural or synthetic) to replace the loss of natural hormones produced by various glands.

HYPOTHALAMUS - A major control centre situated at the base of the brain, regulating body temperature, thirst, appetite and other hormonal glands. It releases hormones that travel directly to the pituitary gland via a stalk.

HYSTERECTOMY - Surgical removal of the uterus.

IMMUNE SYSTEM - The defence and surveillance system of the body, which protects against infection by micro-organisms and invasion by foreign proteins.

IMPLANT - A chemical substance, hormone or object that is surgically implanted into the body.

INFLAMMATION - A condition characterised by swelling, redness, heat and pain in any tissue as a result of trauma, irritation, infection or imbalances in immune function.

LAPAROSCOPE - A long, thin telescopic instrument utilising a fiberoptic lighting system that is inserted through a 1cm incision in the abdominal wall. It functions like a hollow flashlight enabling the surgeon to view internal organs and insert operating instruments through its hollow bore.

LIBIDO - Level of sexual desire.

LUTEINISING HORMONE (LH) - A hormone produced by the pituitary gland, which acts on the ovary to cause ovulation and the production of progesterone.

MALE HORMONE - A hormone, which promotes masculine characteristics in the body, such as facial and body hair, balding, acne, deepening of the voice and increased libido.

MALIGNANT - Cancerous

MANIC DEPRESSION - A mental illness characterised by episodes of euphoric and delusional hyperactivity alternating with deep depressions.

MENOPAUSE - A final cessation of menstruation. The last period.

MENSTRUAL CLOCK - A specialised part of the hypothalamus regulating the cyclical timing of menstrual bleeding.

MENSTRUAL CYCLE - The period of time from the first day of menstruation to the first day of the next menstruation.

MENSTRUATION - Monthly bleeding from the vagina in women of child bearing age, caused by shedding of the lining of the womb.

METABOLIC RATE - The rate at which the body converts food energy into kinetic energy.

METABOLISM - Chemical processes utilising the raw materials of nutrients, oxygen and vitamins along with enzymes, to produce energy for bodily functions.

MICROSURGICAL TECHNIQUES - Surgery performed on small parts of the body such as nerve fibres, blood vessels or fallopian tubes, requiring the use of the operating microscope.

NATUROPATHIC MEDICINE - The treatment of illness with naturally occurring substances such as organic foods, juices, nutritional supplements and herbs.

NEURO-TRANSMITTERS - Chemicals and hormones that transmit messages between the cells and nervous pathways of the brain.

NON-ANDROGENIC - Not causing masculine effects in the body.

OESTRADIOL - A natural oestrogen made by the ovaries. It is the most potent of all the natural oestrogens.

OESTROGENS - Female sex hormones secreted by the ovary, being responsible for the female characteristics of breasts, feminine curves and menstruation. The ovary produces three different types of oestrogen, namely Oestradiol, Oestrone and Oestriol.

ORAL - Denoting a drug to be taken by mouth

ORGASM - The physical and emotional culmination of the sexual act

OSTEOPOROSIS - Loss of bone mass due to loss of bone minerals. Skeletal atrophy. Porous condition of bones.

OVARIAN BLOOD SUPPLY - The blood carried to the ovaries via the ovarian arteries, which branch off from the uterine blood vessels. The ovarian arteries run alongside the fallopian tubes.

OVARIES - The female sex glands (gonads) located on each side of the uterus, which produce eggs and the female sex hormones (oestrogen and progesterone).

OVULATION - The release of the egg from the ovary occurring around mid-cycle.

OVULATION PAIN - Pain occurring at ovulation, which may be sharp and severe and last from a few minutes up to 12 hours.

PELVIC INFLAMMATORY DISEASE (PID) - Inflammation of the pelvic organs, particularly the uterus and fallopian tubes, caused by infectious micro-organisms.

PESSARY - An oval shaped suppository containing drugs or hormones designed to be inserted into the vagina.

PHYSIOLOGICAL - Consistent with the normal functioning of an organism.

PITUITARY GLAND - A mushroom-shaped gland connected by a vascular stalk to the base of the brain. The pituitary gland manufactures hormones, which in turn control other hormonal glands, such as the thyroid, adrenals, ovaries, testicles and breasts.

PLACENTA - The hormonal organ formed in the lining of the uterus by the union of the uterine mucous membrane with the membranes of the foetus to provide for the nourishment of the foetus and the elimination of its waste products.

POLYCYSTIC OVARIAN SYNDROME - A condition of hormonal imbalance characterised by excessive male hormones and irregular menstruation. It is strongly inherited and may be triggered by stress or weight gain.

POLYCYSTIC OVARIES - The type of ovaries present in women with the Polycystic Ovarian Syndrome. They have more than 10 small follicles per ovary aligned around the edge of the ovary, whereas in a 'normal' ovary, they are distributed more evenly throughout the ovary. They can be seen by an ultrasound scan of the pelvis.

POMEROY TECHNIQUE OF TUBAL LIGATION - In this method, the gynae-cologist lifts each fallopian tube to create a loop, ties the base of the loop tightly together with a suture, and cuts off the top of the loop. The suture is gradually absorbed and the two scarred ends of the tube pull apart, leaving a gap between them.

POST-MENOPAUSE - The period of time after the menopause.

POSTNATAL - After childbirth.

POST-PARTUM - After childbirth.

PREMATURE MENOPAUSE - If menopause occurs before the age of 40, it is considered as premature.

PRE-MENOPAUSAL - The years, generally 4 to 5, leading up to the menopause, characterised by a time of hormonal imbalance.

PRE-MENSTRUAL SYNDROME - A collection of variable symptoms, such as mood disturbance, headaches, abdominal bloating, etc, recurring on a cyclical basis in the one to two weeks leading up to menstrual bleeding.

PROGESTOGENS - Synthetic forms of the natural female hormone proges-terone. They are commonly used in the OCP and HRT and regulate men-strual bleeding. Examples are norethisterone, norgestrel and medroxyprog-esterone acetate.

PROGESTERONE ONLY PILL - A contraceptive pill containing only one hor-mone, namely a progesterone such as norethisterone. It is also known as the mini pill.

PROLACTIN - A hormone secreted by the pituitary gland that stimulates milk production in the breasts.

PROSTAGLANDINS -Chemicals manufactured throughout the body, which exert a hormone-like effect and influence muscular contraction, circulation and inflammation.

PSYCHOSIS - A severe mental disorder characterised by delusions, hallucinations, confusion and a breakdown of reality.

PSYCHOSOMATIC - Physical symptoms that are due to psychological and emotional causes and not due to physical disease.

PSYCHOTHERAPY - The treatment of mental and emotional imbalance through analysis of the thought processes, defence mechanisms and subconscious mind.

PSYCHOTIC - A mental illness or patient having the features of a psychosis.

PSYCHOTROPHIC DRUGS - Drugs that act primarily on the brain. Examples are sedatives, tranquillisers and anti-depressants.

PUERPERIUM - The period of time after childbirth required to return the genital organs to their pre-pregnant size and condition. This takes six to eight weeks.

SCAN/ULTRASOUND - See ultrasound.

SEBACEOUS GLANDS - These are tiny oil producing glands in the skin. If they over-produce oil and/or become obstructed, pimples or acne will result.

SEROTONIN - A potent brain chemical, which regulates sleep, mood, libido and appetite.

SEX HORMONES - The male and female hormones produced by the testicles, ovaries, adrenal glands and fat, eg oestrogen, testosterone and progesterone.

STEROID DRUGS AND HORMONES - This group of hormones have a ring-like chemical structure. Examples of steroid hormones are cortisone and the male and female sex hormones.

STROKE - Brain damage resulting from a disturbance of blood supply to the brain.

SYMPTOMS - Physical complaints.

SYNDROME - A group of signs and symptoms that collectively characterise a disease or dysfunction.

SYNERGISTIC NUTRIENT - A nutrient which helps or increases the effect of other body nutrients.

TAILOR-MADE ORAL CONTRACEPTIVE PILL - A pill that is specially designed for you by your doctor to suit your unique physical, mental and contraceptive needs.

TESTOSTERONE - The major male sex hormone.

THYROID GLAND - The endocrine gland situated in front of the neck, which produces the hormone thyroxine.

TRIGLYCERIDES - One of the blood fats, the level of which is influenced by diet, alcohol, exercise and drugs.

TUBAL LIGATION - The surgical obstruction or interruption of the fallopian tubes for the purpose of permanent sterilisation.

TUMOUR - An abnormal growth, which may be cancerous or benign.

UTERUS - The womb.

UROLOGIST - A doctor, who specialises in diseases of the kidneys and urinary tract.

ULTRASOUND SCAN - A method of visualising the internal organs, foetus and blood vessels. Ultrasound does not incur any radiation exposure and utilises very high frequency sound waves (more than 20,000 hertz) that are above the audible limit.

VAGINA - The genital canal or passage leading from the uterus to the vulva; it accommodates the penis during intercourse.

VIRILIZATION - The development of marked masculine physical characteristics.

VULVA - Female external genitalia. Also known as the lips of the vaginal opening.

SUPPORT CONTACTS

Postnatal Depression

www.beyondblue.org.au/postnataldepression/index.aspx

NSW

Karitane: Ph: (02) 9794 1852, Ph: Tollfree 1800 677 961

Tresillian: Ph: (02) 9787 0855, Ph: Tollfree 1800 637 357

ACT

Postnatal and Antenatal Depression Support & Information (PaNDSI)
Ph: (ACT) (02) 6286 4082

QLD

Postnatal Disorders Support Group, Ph: 1300 763 753

Brisbane Centre for Postnatal Disorders, Ph: (07) 3398 0238

VICTORIA

PANDA - Post and Antenatal Depression Association
Phone: (03) 9428 4600, Email: panda@vicnet.net.au

SOUTH AUSTRALIA

Helen Mayo House, Phone (08) 8303 1183

Women's Health Statewide
Ph (08) 8239 9600, Freecall 1800 182 098, Ph 1800 182 098 (TTY)

TASMANIA

Parent Info Telephone Assistance Service, Ph 1800 808 178 (24 hour)

WESTERN AUSTRALIA

Postnatal Depression Support Association, Phone (08) 9340 1622

NORTHERN TERRITORY

Donna Maria Pre and Postnatal Support Network National Helpline
Phone 1300 555 578
Tresillian, Phone Tollfree 1800 637 357

NEW ZEALAND

Lifeline, Ph Auckland (09) 522-2999, Outside Auckland 0800 111-777

REFERENCES

1. Abraham G.E. et al, Hormonal and behavioural changes during the menstrual cycle, Senologia. 1978: 3:33

2. Backstrom CT, et al, Persistence of symptoms of PMT in hysterectomised women, British Journal Obstets & Gynaec. 1981: 88:530

3. Dr Katharina Dalton's original Books (limited availability via amazon.com)
   Once a Month - Understanding & Treating PMS, ISBN = 0897932552
   PMS: The Essential Guide to Treatment Options
   Depression After Childbirth, ISBN = 0192822284
   PMS and Progesterone therapy, Published by Year Book Medical Pub

4. Dalton K, 1970, Brit Med Journal, 2:27

5. Dalton K, 1976, Proceedings Royal Society of Medicine, 59:10, 1014

6. Watson, NR, et al, Gynaec Endocrinol. 4:99-107, 1990

7. Taylor, et al, Current Med Research & Opinion 6, 46-51, 1979

8. Bavernfeind, JC, Vit B6: nutritional & pharmaceutical usage, Pg 78-110, Nat Acad of Sciences, Washington 1978

9. Kerr, GD, Current Med Opinion & Research, Suppl 4, Pg 29, 1977

10. Gordon, T, et al, Am Jour Med. 62: 707, 1977

11. Abrams, AA, New England Journ Med, 272:1080, 1965

12. Abraham G, et al, RBC Magnesium in premenopausal women, International Clinical Nutrition Review, Vol 3, No 1, 1983

13. American Journal of Obstetrics & Gynecology. June 1999 180(6): 1504-11

14. The PEPI Trial; The Post Menopausal Estrogen Progestin Interventions Trial, Effects of HRT on endometrial histology in postmenopausal women, JAMA, 1996, February; 275(5):370-375 and November 276 (17):1430-32 and JAMA 1997, May; 277(19):1515

15. The WHI Study, The Risks & Benefits of Estrogen & Progestin in healthy post-menopausal women, JAMA, Vol 288, No.3, July 17th 2002

16. Wood SH et al, Treatment of premenstrual syndrome with fluoxetine: A double-blind placebo controlled crossover study. Obstet Gynecol 80:339-344, 1992

17. Stone AB et al, Fluoxetine in the treatment of premenstrual syndrome. Psychopharmocol Bull 26:331, 1990

18. Ashby CR, Carr LA, Cook CL, et al: Alteration of platelet serotonin mechanisms and monoamine oxidase activity in premenstrual syndrome. Biol Psychiatry 24:225, 1988.

19. Di Carlo C, Bifulco G, Pellicano M, et al. Hormonal treatment of premenstrual syndrome. Cephalalgia. 1997; 17(Suppl 20):17-9.

20. Brinton LA, et al. Oral contraceptives and breast cancer risk among younger women. Journal of the National Cancer Institute 1995; 87(13): 827835.

Other studies have suggested that there may be an increased risk of developing breast cancer in women who use oral contraceptive pills when they are less than 35 years of age. In a case-control study of women aged 20 through 44 years, 1648 cases of breast cancer and 1505 control subjects were identified.[5] Oral contraceptive pill use for 6 months to 5 years among women less than 45 years of age was associated with a 1.3 relative risk for breast cancer development (95% CI, 1.1 to 1.5). This risk was increased to 1.7 (95% CI, 1.2 to 2.6) in oral contraceptive users less than 35 years of age, with the risk increasing to 2.2 (95% CI, 1.2 to 4.1) in women using the pill more than 10 years and 3.1 (95% CI, 1.4 to 6.7) in women who also began using the pill before age 18. Thus, there is a small but statistically significant relationship between oral contraceptive use and breast cancer in women less than 35 years of age.

21. Schlesselman JJ, Cancer of the breast in relation to OCPs. Contraception 1989; 40(1):1-38

22. Beral V, Results from the Royal College of GPs OCP study, Lancet 1988; 2:131-134

23. Carter JE, et al, J Am Assoc Gynecol Laparosc. 1994 Aug; 1(4, Part 2):S6. Adenomyosis as a Major Cause for Laparoscopic-Assisted Vaginal Hysterectomy for Chronic Pelvic Pain. The possible relationship of adenomyosis to a previous tubal ligation has been explored.

24. De Stefano Long term risk of menstrual disturbance after tubal sterilisation, Am. J. Obstets & Gynec. August 1, 1985, vol 152. no 7, pp835-841

25. Factors seen as links to post tubal ligation syndrome. Contraception Tech. Update Feb 1986, Vol 7, no 2, pp 13-15

26. Cattanach J. Oestrogen deficiency after tubal ligation Lancet April 13, 1985, 1(8433) pp. 847-849

27. Stock, RJ., Sequelae of tubal ligation: An analysis of 75 consecutive hysterectomies. South. Med. J., Oct 1984, Vol. 77, No. 10, pp 1255-1260

28. Cattanach J Post tubal ligation sterilisation problems correlated with ovarian steroidogenesis, Contraception, Nov 1988, vol. 38, No. 5

29. Templeton AA, Hysterectomy following sterilisation, British Journal Obstets & Gynaec.; Oct 1982, Vol. 89, No 10, pp 845-888

30. Donnez J, et al, Tubal polyps, epithelial inclusions, and endometriosis after tubal sterilization. Fertil Steril. 1984 Apr; 41(4):564-8.

31. Contempre B, et al, Effect of selenium supplementation on thyroid hormone metabolism in an iodine and selenium deficient population. Clin Endocrinol (Oxf). 1992 Jun; 36(6):579-83.

32. Derumeaux H. et al, Our findings suggest that selenium may protect against goitre. Selenium was related to thyroid echostructure, suggesting it may also protect against autoimmune thyroid disease. Association of selenium with thyroid volume and echostructure in 35- to 60-year-old French adults. Eur J Endocrinol. 2003 Mar; 148(3):309-15.

33. Fertility Sterility 2003;79:1358-1364

34. Akhtar MS, Trial of momordica charantia powder in patients with maturity onset diabetes. Journal of the Pakistan medical association. 1982, 32:106-107

35. Anderson RA et al, elevated intakes of supplemental chromium improve glucose and insulin variables in type 11 diabetics. Diabetes (1997);46:1786-91

36. Strodter D et al, The influence of lipoic acid on metabolism. Diabetic Res. Clin. Prac. (1995) 29(1):19-26

37. Margaret Rayman, Dietary selenium; time to act, British Medical Journal, Vol. 314, Feb 1997

38. Brown KM, Arthur JR. Selenium, selenoproteins and human health: A Review. Public Health Nutrition, 2001 Apr; 4(2B):593, University of Aberdeen, Scotland. (k.m.brown@abdn.ac.uk)

39. Medina D. et al, Selenium-mediated inhibition mouse mammary tumorigenesis. Cancer Lett 1980;8:241-5

40. Schrauzer. Selenium and Cancer. Bioinorg Chem 1976;5:275

Can't Lose Weight?

Hormones out of balance?

When you've tried everything and nothing seems to work, it's time to visit the specialists at Dr Sandra Cabot's clinics. See a weight loss consultant who is fully qualified in nutrition and natural therapies.

And/or

See a doctor who uses natural bio-identical hormones

Your program includes:

- A detailed dietary and medical history
- Testing of your hormones and metabolism to pin point your exact problem
- A tailor made diet plan based on the results of your blood test
- Ongoing weekly visits with your personal consultant

Assessing emotional and lifestyle issues that may be the barrier between you and weight loss. We dedicate ourselves to seeing you through your weight loss from start to finish.

Our program is designed to check for **ALL** the hidden obstacles to weight loss, including hormonal and metabolic imbalances.

At a cost so competitive, that we guarantee you won't be able to put a better price on your health.

Compounding Pharmacy	Suburb	State	Phone
AINSLIE PHARMACY	AINSLIE	ACT	02 6248 7708
APPIN PHARMACY	APPIN	NSW	02 46311488
ASHGROVE DAY & NIGHT PHARMACY	ASHGROVE	QLD	07 3366 1740
ASPLEY MEDICAL CENTRE CHEMIST	ASPLEY	QLD	07 3263 1957
AUSTRALIAN CUSTOM PHARMACEUTIC	TAREN POINT	NSW	02 8536 4100
AUSTRALIAN PHARMACY COMPOUNDIN	BANKSTOWN	NSW	02 9793 1161
BALHANNAH JUNCTION PHARMACY	BALHANNAH	SA	08 8388 4721
BELGIAN GARDEN'S PHARMACY	TOWNSVILLE	QLD	074771 5565
BELLAMBI PHARMACY	BELLAMBI	NSW	02 4227 3171
BELVEDERE PARK PHARMACY	SEAFORD	VIC	03 9786 2703
BIO PHARM	CURRUMBIN WATERS	QLD	07 5598 6409
BOB HARRISON SP CHEMIST	MIRANDA	NSW	02 9524 7131
CARILLON MEDICAL CENTRE PHARMA	NEWTOWN	NSW	02 9519 4247
CARINA DAY & NIGHT PHARMACY	CARINA	QLD	07 3398 2501
CASTLEREAGH PHARMACY	SYDNEY	NSW	02 9261 3664
CASULA MALL SOUL PATTINSON	CASULA	NSW	02 9821 1323
CHEMMART WINDSOR PHARMACY	WINDSOR	QLD	07 3857 5666
CHITTAWAY PHARMACY	CHITTAWAY	NSW	02 4388 4722
CINCOTTA CHEMIST	MERRYLANDS	NSW	02 9897 1011
CLAYTON CHEM MART PHARMACY	CLAYTON	VIC	03 9544 3644
COMPOUNDIA	DOCK LANDS	VIC	03 9670 2882
CRANE'S PHARMACIST ADVICE	FORSTER	NSW	02 6555 5589
DALLIMORES PHARMACY	PERTH	WA	08 9228-0224
DARTNELL'S PHARMACY	SURREY HILLS	VIC	03 9888 5899
DEE WHY HEALTH CARE PHARMACY	DEE WHY	NSW	02 9971 5353
DENNIS HAM AMCAL PHARMACY	WARRNAMBOOL	VIC	03 5562 9780
DOVE'S PHARMACY	KALLAROO	WA	08 9307 4555
DUPUY'S PHARMACY	MACKAY	QLD	07 4942 3274
DURAL VILLAGE SOUL PATTINSON	DURAL	NSW	02 9651 3547
EASTLAKES PHARMACY	EASTLAKES	NSW	02 9667 2570
EASTPOINT SOUL PATTINSON PHARM	EDGECLIFF	NSW	02 9328 1316
EMSLIES FLOREAT PHARMACY	FLOREAT	WA	08 9387 1803
ENGADINE D&N PHARMACY	ENGADINE	NSW	02 9520 8838
EVERYDAY FAMILY CHEMIST	WOLLONGONG	NSW	02 4226 3188
FOUNTAIN GATE	MELBOURNE	VIC	03 9705 7133
FRESH THERAPEUTICS	BROADWAY, SYDNEY	NSW	02 9281 6816
FURLEY'S PHARMACY	DOUBLE BAY	NSW	02 9327 5871
GAVIN STARR PHARMACIST	LANE COVE	NSW	02 9427 1755
GLENHUNTLY PHARMACY	GLENHUNTLY	VIC	03 95715290
GOODHEALTH PHARMACIES	CLAYFIELD	QLD	07 3262 3517
GOODING DRIVE PHAMACY	CARRARA	QLD	07 55305888
HAYBOROUGH PHARMACY	HAYBOROUGH	SA	0412 187 423
HIGH ST PHARMACY	WILLOUGHBY	NSW	02 9958 8153
HUNTER CONNECT PHARMACY	SYDNEY	NSW	02 9235 0406
HYNES PHARMACY	BUNDABERG	QLD	07 4151 3016
JEWELLSTOWN AMCAL PHARMACY	JEWELLSTOWN	NSW	02 4948 5766
JIM GREEN'S PHARMACY	GEELONG	VIC	03 5229 3539
JIMBOOMBA PHARMACY	JIMBOOMBA	QLD	07 5546 9555
JOHN HALPIN PHARMACY	LISMORE	NSW	1800 243 6478
JOZEF TJONG	HORNSBY	NSW	0422 285 366
KEILOR DOWNS CARING CHEMIST	KEILOR DOWNS	VIC	03 9367 6133
KINGSFORD CHEMIST	KINGSFORD	NSW	02 9663 3900
KINGSWAY MEDICAL CENTRE PHARMA	DEE WHY	NSW	02 9982 6383

KOZANOGLU PHARMACY	COBURG	VIC	03 9383 5518
LADHOPE PHARMACY	BRISBANE	QLD	07 3831 5762
LATROBE UNIVERSITY	BENDIGO	VIC	03 5444 7383
LIFELINE HEALTH PHARMACY	TRARALGON	VIC	03 5174 2003
LINCOLN DISPENSARY	WEST PERTH	WA	08 9321 3312
LORRAINE MORONEY	MASCOT	NSW	02 9667 4144
MACQUARIE PHARMACY	MACQUARIE	ACT	02 6251 1063
MACREADIE'S TEWANTIN	TEWANTIN	QLD	07 5449 7899
MAIN STREET PHARMACY	OSBORNE PARK	WA	08 93443040
MARION CHEMPLUS	MARION	SA	08 8276 8600
MATER PHARMACY SERVICES	SOUTH BRISBANE	QLD	07 3840 8922
MAWSON PHARMACY	MAWSON	ACT	02 6286 3737
MAYLANDS 7 DAY PHARMACY	MAYLANDS	WA	08 9370 4410
MAZZEI'S PHARMACY	EASTWOOD	NSW	02 9874 1547
MELBOURNE CENTRE	SEDDON	VIC	03 9689 0833
MERCY PHARMACY	MT LAWLEY	WA	08 9371 9119
MORPHETT VALE CHEMMART	MORPHETT VALE	SA	08 8382 3300
MOSMAN PHARMACY	MOSMAN	NSW	02 9969 6194
NATIONWIDE PHARMACY	CAULFIELD SOUTH	VIC	03 9532 8555
NEW HORIZONS PHARMACY	BALMAIN	NSW	02 98185822
NORANDA CHEMMART PHARMACY	NORANDA	WA	08 9375 1251
OPTIMUS HEALTHCARE	NEWMARKET AUCKLAND	NZ	00116495200022
PETER ALLAN	MOUNT VICTORIA	NSW	02 98084830
PETER COOK AMCAL	TUART HILL	WA	08 9349 1065
PHARMACEUTICAL NZ	AUCKLAND	NZ	0011 64 9 480 2660
PHARMACY 777 APPLECROSS	APPLECROSS	WA	08 9364 8777
PHARMACY HELP MANDURAH	MANDURAH	WA	08 9581 4833
PHARMACYSMART PHARMACY	DONCASTER	VIC	03 9848 2001
PINDARA PHARMACY	BEWOWA	QLD	07 5539 2000
PITTWATER PHARMACY	MONAVALE	NSW	02 9999 3398
POORAKA CHEMPLUS	POORAKA	SA	08 8262 3949
RAJU'S PHARMACY	GISBORNE	VIC	03 5428 2107
REINKE'S PHARMACY	TOOWOOMBA	QLD	07 46324534
RICHARD STENLAKE CHEMIST	BONDI JUNCTION	NSW	02 9387 3205
SHIRLEY JAMES PHARMACY	STRATHFIELDSAYE	VIC	03 5439 3513
SINGLETON HEIGHTS PHARMACY	SINGLETON HEIGHTS	NSW	02 6573 1410
SKYLINE PHARMACY	FRENCHS FOREST	NSW	02 9451 4169
SOUTH MELBOURNE PHARMACY	SOUTH MELBOURNE	VIC	03 9690 5240
SINGAPORE COMPOUNDING CENTRE	1 ORCHARD BVD		0011 65 6836 1323
ST QUENTINS AMCAL	CLAREMONT	WA	08 9383 1826
TERREY HILLS DAY & NIGHT PHARM	TERREY HILLS	NSW	02 9450 1768
THE GREEN DISPENSARY COMPOUNDING	ERINDALE	SA	08 8431 6727
THE GROVE	NEUTRAL BAY	NSW	02 9953 5506
THOMPSONS AMCAL CHEMIST	ELTHAM	VIC	03 9439 9695
TONI RILEY PHARMACIES	BENDIGO	VIC	03 5443 5233
TUCKERS PHARMACY	RAMSGATE	NSW	02 9529 7472
TUGUN CHEMMART CHEMIST	TUGUN	QLD	07 5534 2327
VISIONARY HEALTH COMPOUNDING	HAMILTON	NSW	02 4969 5081
WAL'S PHARMACY	WARILLA	NSW	02 4295 1429
WALKER ST PHARMACY	NORTH SYDNEY	NSW	02 9955 5691
WALSH'S VILLAGE PHARMACY	MAROUBRA	NSW	02 9311 0088
WEST LINDFIELD PHARMACY	LINDFIELD	NSW	02 9416 2642
WESTMEADOWS PHARMACY	WESTMEADOWS	VIC	03 9338 4894
WICKHAM HOUSE PHARMACY	BRISBANE	QLD	07 3831 5847
YANDINA PHARMACY	YANDINA	QLD	07 5446 7989